www.harcourt-internat

Bringing you products from all Harcourt [...] companies including Baillière Tindall, Chu[...] Livingstone, Mosby and W.B. Saunders

D1760613

Dr Ahmed Iqbal

○ **Browse** for latest information on new books, journals and electronic products

○ **Search** for information on over 20 000 published titles with full product information including tables of contents and sample chapters

○ **Keep up to date** with our extensive publishing programme in your field by registering with eAlert or requesting postal updates

○ **Secure online ordering** with prompt delivery, as well as full contact details to order by phone, fax or post

○ **News** of special features and promotions

If you are based in the following countries, please visit the country-specific site to receive full details of product availability and local ordering information

USA: www.harcourthealth.com

Canada: www.harcourtcanada.com

Australia: www.harcourt.com.au

Baillière Tindall   CHURCHILL LIVINGSTONE   Mosby   W.B. SAUNDERS

Pass the
MR(

(Part

All the -   ou need

Pass the MRCS

(Parts I and II)

All the techniques you need

Alison Walker
Chris Macklin
Christopher Williams

Foreword By
Professor M J McMahon

W.B. Saunders Company Ltd

EDINBURGH LONDON NEW YORK PHILADELPHIA ST LOUIS SYDNEY TORONTO 2001

W.B. SAUNDERS
An imprint of Harcourt Publishers Limited

© Harcourt Publishers Limited 2001

 is a registered trademark of Harcourt Publishers Limited

The right of Alison Walker, Chris Macklin and Christopher Williams to be identified as authors of this work has been asserted by them in accordance with the Copyright, Designs and Patents Act 1988

First published 2001

ISBN 070202578X

British Library Cataloguing in Publication Data
A catalogue record for this book is available from the British Library

Library of Congress Cataloging in Publication Data
A catalog record for this book is available from the Library of Congress

Note
Medical knowledge is constantly changing. As new information becomes available, changes in treatment, procedures, equipment and the use of drugs become necessary. The authors and the publishers have taken care to ensure that the information given in this text is accurate and up-to-date. However, readers are strongly advised to confirm that the information, especially with regard to drug usage, complies with the latest legislation and standards of practice.

The
publisher's
policy is to use
**paper manufactured
from sustainable forests**

Printed in China

Contents

MRCS Part II – the clinical exams

Authors and contributors

Authors

Miss Alison Walker
Specialist Registrar in Accident and Emergency, Leeds General Infirmary, Leeds, UK

Mr Chris Macklin
Specialist Registrar in General Surgery, Yorkshire Region, UK

Dr Christopher Williams
Senior Lecturer/Honorary Consultant in Psychiatry, Department of Psychological Medicine, Gartnavel Royal Hospital, Glasgow, UK

Contributors

Dr Kevin Appleton
Consultant in Child and Adolescent Psychiatry, Marinoto West, Waitakere Hospital, Auckland, New Zealand

Dr Keith Brownlee
Consultant Paediatrician, St. James's University Hospital, Leeds, UK

Dr Siân McIver
Specialist Registrar in Forensic Psychiatry, Fieldhead Hospital, Wakefield, UK

Dr David Protheroe
Consultant in Liaison Psychiatry, Leeds General Infirmary, Leeds, UK

Dr Peter Trigwell
Consultant in Liaison Psychiatry, Department of Liaison Psychiatry, Leeds, UK

Dr David Yeomans
Consultant Psychiatrist, Overthorpe House, Leeds, UK

The structure of this book and some material is based on others in the 'Pass the...' series, published by W B Saunders, with kind permission of the authors.

Foreword

Ever since I qualified in medicine I have encountered books telling me how to pass this or that exam. Some were valuable, some less so. The common feature which most of them shared was that they were really textbooks containing subject matter presented in a particular format which it was hoped would help the candidate to pass the exam. In most cases he or she would be better to read a standard authoritative text on the subject.

'Pass the MRCS' is different. This book does not contain any surgical subject matter, but is a compilation of advice and guidance to help those about to sit Parts I and II of the MRCS examination. This is especially useful at the present time because the transition from FRCS to MRCS has left some candidates a little confused and concerned about the new exams.

This book provides valuable information about the examinations of the different surgical colleges which will help candidates to select the examination they wish to sit and to obtain information about the timings of the exam and when to apply for it.

It is written by two surgeons and a psychiatrist (it is probably necessary for anybody contemplating surgical exams to see a psychiatrist) and provides insight into the general approaches to the examination as well as specific details about the individual parts of the exams. The candidates who read this book when commencing a surgical career will be able to plan their work, the timing of their applications for the exam and their approach to it in a logical and, hopefully, relaxed manner. I'm sure it will contribute greatly to a reduction in the level of anxiety which I personally experienced in sitting the old style primary and fellowship examinations.

Professor M J McMahon,
ChM, PhD, FRCS
Professor of Surgery, Leeds General Infirmary, Leeds, UK

Introduction

Clinical competence and passing the Membership Examinations for the Royal Colleges of Surgeons are the most visible criteria by which trainees progress up the career ladder in any branch of surgery. Taking the exams is costly in both financial and personal terms. To pass requires very significant work and commitment. The aim of this book is to provide a concise guide to all parts of the MRCS exam, and is the first book of its kind which focuses on the important area of exam techniques. **N.B.** For simplicity the term MRCS is used to mean Membership of the Royal College of Surgeons of Edinburgh, the Royal College of Surgeons of England, the Royal College of Physicians and Surgeons of Glasgow or the Royal College of Surgeons in Ireland (which awards the Associate Fellowship of the Royal College of Surgeons in Ireland, AFRCSI).

This book is not a 'crammer' book of key facts for the exam. You will find that very few factual pieces of information are presented. Instead, it will help you to present the information that you have learned elsewhere (whether from formal revision, everyday clinical practice or other sources) in a professional and structured way. Even very good clinicians with a strong factual knowledge may fail the exams because of poor technique. This book will help you to use your knowledge and experience effectively to enable you to pass. At the same time we hope to help you develop the skills of a good clinician: someone who can manage their time, think quickly and efficiently, and present themselves professionally in exam and interview situations.

The book is divided into sections:
- Preparing for the MRCS exam
- MRCS Part I – the MCQ exams
- MRCS Part II – the clinical exams

We hope that you will find our book helpful. In producing any book such as this, many other people are always involved. In particular we would like to thank Professor Michael McMahon, who wrote the foreword, and those who have reviewed the book and suggested improvements. Finally, we wish to thank our families and colleagues who have supported us during the writing of the book.

Alison Walker
Chris Macklin
Christopher Williams
July 2000

Preparing for the exam

Important practical and preparation issues

Introduction

If you wish to pursue a career in any surgical specialty it will be necessary for you to pass the exams that lead on to Membership of the Royal College of Surgeons (MRCS). It is very unlikely that you will get a place on a surgical rotation without the Membership. Additionally, in many countries in the world the MRCS is highly regarded as a measure of clinical competence and in some countries, as in the British Isles, it is a hurdle which has to be successfully negotiated on the way to becoming a specialist. The exams are organized by the four Royal Colleges:

- The Royal College of Surgeons of England
- The Royal College of Surgeons of Edinburgh
- The Royal College of Physicians and Surgeons of Glasgow
- The Royal College of Surgeons in Ireland.

Although we have provided a basic outline of the examination format for each College, you should obtain – and read – the examination regulations and information for candidates, which are available from all the Royal Colleges (addresses, telephone numbers and websites are at the end of this chapter). You should read them particularly carefully if your career has been unusual in any way or if you are applying from abroad.

Examination format

The examination consists of three parts – the multiple choice questions (MCQs) of Part I, and the clinicals and vivas of Part II.

These are consistent between the Colleges but the exact format of the examinations varies. The Colleges have reciprocity with regard to Part I and all require similar types of Basic Surgical Training (BST) posts to be completed prior to application. Each College has specific requirements relating to how much time you have been in approved training in order for you to be eligible to sit the exam. It is essential that candidates obtain the current requirements from the relevant College as these change from time to time. Each Royal College requires a logbook to be submitted for each post completed as part of the exam.

The marking method for the MCQ examinations differs among the colleges and is either **negative** or **neutral**. Because the strategy for answering MCQs is very different for negatively- and neutrally-marked papers, we have summarized the essential MCQ techniques appropriate for both marking styles in Chapter 3.

The following summarizes the different requirements of the Colleges as of January 2000. Many Royal Colleges, however, are currently reviewing their membership exams in order to improve their structure and content. You should always request up-to-date details of the exam, both to identify the different components and to help you to focus your revision.

The Royal College of Surgeons of England

Basic requirements

Candidates need to complete 24 months in BST (Basic Surgical Training), including two 6-month posts in accident and emergency, general surgery or orthopaedics. The other 12 months can include 6-month posts in cardiothoracic surgery, neurosurgery, oral and maxillofacial surgery, ear nose and throat (ENT), paediatric surgery, plastic surgery, urology, gynaecology or ophthalmology. Credit will be given for up to 4 months in an Intensive Therapy Unit (ITU) post and accident and emergency, orthopaedics or general surgery can be included if they have not been undertaken previously.

Completion of a 'Basic Surgical Skills' course is compulsory and the College advises candidates to undertake an 'Advanced Trauma Life Support' (ATLS) course and a 'Care of the Critically Ill Surgical Patient'course.

Components of the exam

MCQs
The MCQs may be taken at any time in a 24-month BST programme. They are held biannually in London and at regional centres. The two papers can be taken in any order, separately or together. Each paper will be awarded a 'Pass' or 'Fail' and only failed papers need to be retaken.

Paper	Number of questions	Time allowed
MCQ 1: Core Modules	300	2 hours
MCQ 2: System Modules	300	2 hours

The MCQs are **neutrally marked** (i.e. one mark is added for each correct answer and no marks are given for incorrect or omitted answers). There is no limit to the number of times a candidate may attempt the MCQs.

The clinical exam
Held biannually in London and at regional centres. Candidates must have passed the MCQ section. The clinical exam can be taken after completion of 20 months of BST. The clinical comprises a series of **short cases completed over 1 hour**. The candidate examines patients in five bays.
The bays are entitled:

- Superficial lesions
- Musculoskeletal and neurosurgery
- Circulatory and lymphatic
- Trunk
- Communication skills.

Marks are allocated equally in each bay.

The vivas

Held biannually in London. Candidates must have passed the MCQ and clinical sections and have completed 22 months of BST. Questions may cover the whole syllabus and are asked during three vivas.

Viva	Time allowed
Viva 1: Applied Surgical Anatomy and Operative Surgery	20 minutes
Viva 2: Applied Physiology and Critical Care	20 minutes
Viva 3: Clinical Pathology and Principles of Surgery	20 minutes

NB   Surgical logbooks are required at the clinical and viva examinations.

The clinical and viva sections must be completed successfully within 2 years of first attempting the clinical section.

The Royal College of Surgeons of Edinburgh

Basic requirements

Candidates need to complete 24 months in BST, with 12 months spent in 6-month posts in accident and emergency, general surgery or orthopaedics. The other 12 months can include 6-month posts in cardiothoracic surgery, neurosurgery, oral and maxillofacial surgery, ENT, paediatric surgery, plastic surgery or urology. Credit will be given for up to 4 months in an ITU post. Accident and emergency, orthopaedics or general surgery can be included if they have not been undertaken previously.

Completion of a Basic Surgical Skills course is compulsory and the College advises candidates to undertake an ATLS course.

Components of the exam

MCQs
The MCQ papers may be taken at any time in the BST period. There is no limit to the number of times each paper can be taken.

Paper		Number of questions	Time allowed
MCQ 1:	Principles of Surgery in General	300	2 hours
MCQ 2:	Specialist Subjects	300	2 hours

The pass mark is 140/300 and the paper is **negatively marked** (i.e. one mark is added for each correct answer, no marks are awarded for a 'don't know' or omitted response, and one mark is subtracted for each incorrect response).

Candidates can apply for the final assessment exams (Part II) after 18 months of BST. The *clinicals*, however, cannot be taken until 20 months of BST have been completed.

The vivas

Viva		Time allowed
Viva 1:	Critical Care	20 minutes
Viva 2:	Principles of Surgery including Operative Surgery and Applied Anatomy (this may include photographs, imaging, pathological specimens etc.)	20 minutes
Viva 3:	Clinical Surgery and Pathology (logbook-based)	20 minutes

The clinical exam
At least five cases will be covered in 40 minutes. The exam is used to assess the ability to take a concise history, assess physical signs, formulate a differential diagnosis, and identify appropriate investigations and treatment. Candidates need to achieve a minimum mark in the vivas in order to proceed to the clinicals. If you sit both clinicals and vivas and only pass one, you need only resit the failed part.

The Royal College of Physicians and Surgeons of Glasgow

Basic requirements

Candidates need to complete 24 months in BST, including two 6-month posts in accident and emergency, general surgery or orthopaedics. The other 12 months can include 6-month posts in cardiothoracic surgery, neurosurgery, oral and maxillofacial surgery, ENT, paediatric surgery, plastic surgery, urology, gynaecology or ophthalmology. Credit will be given for up to 4 months in an ITU post. Accident and emergency, orthopaedics or general surgery posts can be included if they have not been undertaken previously.

Completion of a Basic Surgical Skills course is compulsory.

Components of the exam

MCQs
The format of the MCQs was changed in 1999 from four 1-hour papers to two 2-hour papers. These can be taken at any time during BST.

Paper		Number of questions	Time allowed
Paper 1:	Core Modules	90	2 hours
Paper 2:	System Modules	90	2 hours

The MCQs are **neutrally marked**.

The vivas

Eighteen months of BST and a Basic Surgical Skills course must have been completed before applying for the vivas.

Viva	Time allowed
Viva 1: Applied Anatomy, Operative Surgery, Principles and Practice of Surgery	30 minutes
Viva 2: Applied Pathology/Bacteriology, Critical Care/Surgical Pathology	30 minutes

The clinical exam

Candidates must pass the vivas before they can sit the clinical exam. The clinical exam consists of a **40-minute ward round** of **a minimum of five patients**: you will have to elicit a history, interpret clinical signs, and discuss investigations and treatment. The clinical exams must be passed within 2 years of the first attempt at the clinical section. If both the clinical and the viva are attempted and only one is passed, the candidate need only resit the failed part.

The Royal College of Surgeons in Ireland

Basic requirements

Candidates need to complete 24 months in BST, including two 6-month posts in accident and emergency, general surgery or orthopaedics. The other 12 months can include 6-month posts in cardiothoracic surgery, neurosurgery, oral and maxillofacial surgery, ENT, paediatric surgery, plastic surgery, urology or ophthalmology. Credit will be given for up to 4 months in an ITU post. Accident and emergency, orthopaedics or general surgery can be included if they were not undertaken previously.

Completion of a Basic Surgical Skills course is compulsory and candidates are advised to attend an ATLS course.

Components of the exam

MCQs

The MCQs may be taken at any time during BST. The exam consists of four 1-hour papers. Each paper has 20 questions, which have five stems each, making a total of **100 questions per paper**.

Paper	Number of questions	Time allowed
Paper 1: Surgical Anatomy	20 (〈 5)	1 hour
Paper 2: Surgical Pathology	20 (〈 5)	1 hour
Paper 3: Applied Pathology Microbiology and Immunology	20 (〈 5)	1 hour
Paper 4: Clinical Surgery	20 (〈 5)	1 hour

A total mark of 240/500 must be attained to pass the MCQ section. The MCQs are **neutrally marked**.

The vivas

Taken after a minimum of 18 months of BST.

Viva	Time allowed
Viva 1: Operative Surgery and Surgical Anatomy	30 minutes
Viva 2: Critical Care and Surgical Emergencies	30 minutes
Viva 3: Principles of Surgical Management	30 minutes

Each viva is marked out of 100 and candidates must score 180/300 to pass.

The clinical exam

This part of the exam may be attempted after 21 months of BST and consists of **a minimum of five cases in 1 hour**. The clinical exams must be passed within 2 years of the first attempt at the clinical section. The format includes history-taking, patient examination and the interpretation of clinical signs.

> **Important Note**: The above descriptions of the Royal College examinations are current at the time of writing. However, all exams are prone to change and you should obtain the up-to-date exam details from your chosen Royal College.

Applying to sit the exams

Places are limited at all examination centres and it is therefore advisable to apply early. You must request application forms from the College and submit these on time with the appropriate fee, payable in pounds sterling. The deadline is surprisingly early and you need to request the application forms several months in advance. It is not uncommon for candidates to 'miss the boat'– book early to avoid disappointment and increased stress.

Preparation

- Once you have decided when to take the exam, immediately work out a timetable for revision. This can be detailed or simply a broad outline, depending on your preference. Try to mix subjects you find easy with more difficult areas and maintain variety and interest. Be flexible as you work through your revision. If there are areas in which you are struggling, spend a bit more time on these and a bit less on those areas in which you are confident. **The revision timetable must be realistic and achievable**. A timetable can inspire increased motivation to work, as you can see what needs to be done and what areas have been covered. It will also help to keep you on target for the exam.

- Most people assign a period of 3–6 months each for revision for Parts I and II. Others may prefer a relatively shorter period of intense 'cramming'. This may be stressful and most people find that it is more helpful to work consistently (e.g. 2 hours a night), but be flexible to allow for relaxation, on-call commitments and other occasions. You have to decide which approach suits you best.
- Many candidates find it helpful to decide on a day each week when they will definitely not revise. Having **regular breaks** helps to maintain commitment the rest of the time. Remember to continue to enjoy some social activities: these will be a useful antidote to your revision.
- Following one of the major textbooks may help to structure your revision timetable. You will need a checklist of subject areas to ensure that you cover everything required. It is useful to build up a selection of 'stock' answers for the clinical and oral exams.
- **Consider going on an examination course early in your revision**, rather than going just before the exam. The advantage of doing this is that the course can help you get a 'feel' for what is required and may highlight potentially weak areas.
- **Do not burn yourself out or peak too early**. Your preparations should be like those of an athlete getting ready for an important race: increase the tempo as the exams approach, but keep something in reserve for the final weeks. Do not arrive at the exam feeling stale, jaded and having lost interest.

Practice

An analysis of your learning style, as described in Chapter 2, will shape the way you prepare for the exams. For *every* candidate practice is essential. It is important to **test yourself regularly** throughout the revision period in order to get feedback on your performance. This will identify stronger and weaker areas, help you to focus your revision and practise on weaker areas.

For Part I you will need to practise MCQs. For Part II you will need to practise answering questions on case histories and on clinical material. For Part II you must practise *both* parts of the exam. Candidates too often concentrate only on the short cases because these are perceived to be the most difficult part of the exam and because they lend themselves most easily to teaching sessions. Both parts of the exam are important and you should ensure that you are familiar with each component.

Ask your peers and senior colleagues to listen to your presentations and give you feedback. Think critically about their comments but do not take them too much to heart. Each person you ask will have a slightly different opinion on what is good and bad about your efforts. Focus on what you find to be most helpful and try to make changes based on the balance of what has been said. With adequate practice you will have built up confidence in your abilities before you enter the examination room.

The benefits of addressing your exam technique

Good preparation and adequate practice will enable you to feel confident that the exam is not going to bring too many surprises. It should also prevent you from being thrown off-balance by a difficult question, or at least enable you to function on 'autopilot' until you regain your equilibrium. You should have prepared answers and answering techniques for difficult questions. You should know how to impress examiners with your presentation technique. You should know the details of the exam structure, how it is marked and what is expected of you. This will help to reduce your anxiety and improve your exam performance.

Your mental health

Examinations cause stress over an extended period. It is worthwhile to consider how the process is affecting you. Do you need a break? What about a holiday or a night out? What about relaxation, sport and television? If you do suffer from exam nerves it pays to practise relaxation beforehand. It takes time to learn these skills – buying a relaxation tape the week before the exam is unlikely to be as useful as learning the skills over several weeks or months. Do this for your mock exams too.

Last-minute revision is sometimes more of an anxiolytic than an aid to memory: do it if you *have* to, but a day of rest before the exams can be therapeutic. Lastly, although some people have been known to find anxiolytics or beta-blockers helpful, medication should generally be avoided.

State of mind on the exam day

In order to do well in the exams it helps not to be distracted. Some find it easy to concentrate but others may need to focus actively on the exam. Try to exclude unhelpful thoughts of work, home and low confidence. Practise relaxation techniques if these helped during revision. Reassure yourself that all your preparation means that you are at an advantage before the exam even starts and that, with luck, you will have already prepared answers to some of the questions that will arise.

Practical issues

- Make it easy on yourself. Get study leave arranged well in advance and stick to it. Consider attending a revision course. It may be helpful to take a week off work just before the exam for final preparations.
- Do not be persuaded to cover for an absent colleague at the last moment: you have spent too much time, effort and money to let personnel issues get in your way. Give yourself at least one clear day off work before travelling to the exam centre.
- If you are staying overnight choose a comfortable hotel in a quiet location – it is worth the money. Do not skimp on last-

minute comforts, especially if you can claim expenses. Ring Personnel in advance to find out what you are entitled to. (Some employers pay for revision courses.) If, when you arrive at the hotel, it is clearly unsuitable (e.g. noisy or dirty), leave it and move elsewhere – a good night's sleep is well worth the cost of better accommodation.

- Give yourself plenty of time to get to the exam centre: it is better to arrive 2 hours early than 2 minutes late. If you are late for any part of the exam you may feel tense and pressured and will be less likely to perform well. This could destroy months of hard work and you might have to repeat all your revision once again.
- If using public transport consider a back-up route in case the service is disrupted. In general, if you leave early enough you will be able to cope with traffic and rail delays. Consider flying longer distances. Pack in advance and do not rush.
- In the clinical exam your personal presentation will earn marks. Dress appropriately. Be polite and courteous to everyone.

After the exam

You will not know for certain how things have gone, though you may feel elated or depressed at your performance. Parts of the exam leave the vast majority of candidates thinking that they have probably failed (although many have passed). These feelings may continue for some time. Try to avoid too many post-mortems: going over your answers again and again in your mind, analysing possible mistakes, is rarely helpful. A holiday break away may be a good idea.

You have to wait a while for the results, especially for the MCQs. If you pass, well done. If not, then **try again**, as many members and fellows of the Royal Colleges have had to in the past. Take note of the feedback from the examiners and keep working on your exam technique. See Appendix 1: *What if you fail?–Trying again*.

> **Key points**
>
> ✔ Obtain and read the exam regulations and information for candidates.
> ✔ Understand how they apply to you and use the materials to help focus your revision.
> ✔ Practise presentation and examination techniques as well as purely learning facts.
> ✔ When you have decided to take the exam, send off for the application forms early.
> ✔ Submit completed forms, with the appropriate fee, in good time.
> ✔ Formulate a comprehensive revision timetable, including time off for relaxation and recreation.
> ✔ Examination technique can help you communicate what you know to your best ability. Think carefully about this aspect of the exam.
> ✔ Practise each component of the exams again and again to improve your performance.

USEFUL ADDRESSES

The Royal College of Surgeons of England
35–43 Lincoln's Inn Fields
London WC2A 3PN
Tel: 0207 312 6625
Fax: 0207 312 6623
Internet: *www.rcseng.ac.uk*
Application form: *www.rcseng.ac.uk/public/exams/mrcsremain.htm*

The Royal College of Surgeons of Edinburgh
Nicolson Street
Edinburgh EH8 9DW
Tel: 0131 527 1600
Fax: 0131 557 6406
Internet: *www.rcsed.ac.uk*

The Royal College of Physicians and Surgeons of Glasgow
232–242 St Vincent's Street
Glasgow G2 5RJ

Tel: 0141 221 6072
Fax: 0141 221 1804
Internet: *www.rcpsglasg.ac.uk*

The Royal College of Surgeons in Ireland
123 St Stephen's Green
Dublin 2
Eire
Tel: + 353 1 402 2100
Internet: *www.rcsi.ie*
Application form:
www.rcsi.ie/postgrad_education/examinations/application.html

2

Learning styles and revision strategies

Introduction

It is often believed that success in medical examinations simply depends on faithful regurgitation of facts. This is not the whole truth. It is possible to know the facts of a subject very well and still fail the examination. You *can* improve your exam performance significantly, however, with good technique. **Technique refers to your style of learning and preparing, and of using and presenting the learnt information to best effect**.

Membership examinations are complex and difficult. It may be some time since you have taken a major examination or worked in the way required to prepare for such a challenge. During house jobs you may well have taken a break from formal study, choosing instead to develop your practical skills and learn about everyday clinical medicine. The first part of membership tests the breadth of your surgical knowledge. You will need to focus on re-learning the basic sciences again. This is an area you will probably have neglected since the days of your preclinical training. It is, therefore, particularly important to think specifically about learning styles and the way you will go about preparing to sit the exams. You must decide both *what* to learn, and *how* to structure your learning.

Learning styles

Sit back for a moment and consider what you know about how you learn. Do you think that you have a personal learning style? It is very likely that you do, as you have spent at least 20 years in education developing your own methods of study. For example, you probably found that your own lecture notes at university were very different from those of your friends.

The following is a list of questions about learning style. Work through it point by point – it is designed to help you to think about *how* you learn.

- Do you revise in a **suitable environment** (– quiet, warm enough, well lit, with a minimum of disturbance)? How can you **improve** the environment? This may involve choosing to leave the house and work elsewhere (e.g. the library or local academic/postgraduate centre). Candidates who have children may find that some sessions spent away from home (or a period of time such as a week away from home) can be helpful, if this can be agreed with their spouse or partner.
- Do you **focus your learning?** There is no point revising material for the exam that is unlikely to be examined. More importantly, you must not miss out subjects that you will be expected to know about and understand.
- Can you **prioritize** (– learn the common things before the esoteric)?
- Do you **set and achieve your goals** (e.g. to learn the cranial nerves and their branches *today* and ensure that you reach this goal)?
- Do you **review what you have learned** (e.g. use MCQs to test what you have just learned and to identify weak areas that need more work)?
- Do you know what **sources of information** you are most comfortable with? Some people use up-to-date textbooks; others prefer to use a mixture of smaller texts and journal articles. Do not forget to concentrate on the main areas – these can be overlooked if you become bogged down in the fine detail of more obscure topics.
- Do you **keep the exam in mind while learning** (– in order to spot questions, rehearse answers and memorize information in the style appropriate to the exam)?

- **How *much* information** can you take in at one go? There is no point staring at a book when your concentration seems to have gone. Taking short but regular breaks may help you to consolidate what you have learned and maintain your focus.
- **How much repetition** do you need? Does it help to read several accounts from different books, perhaps followed by a re-read of your own notes to fix those facts in your memory? Alternatively, are you the type of person who prefers to learn thoroughly from just one or two books?
- Do you review areas you have already covered? Try to revise the topic again after 1 week and after 4 weeks to check your understanding and memory.
- Do you **use your daily work to help you learn** (e.g. practising your clinical assessments, spending time reflecting on your differential diagnoses and management plans in your normal work)? Do you write up case notes in exam format?
- Are you **adequately motivated**? Try to make your reasons for applying positive (e.g. career progression or self-satisfaction), rather than negative (e.g. 'because I should', the fear of financial loss or 'failure avoidance'). Passing the exam requires prolonged personal commitment and motivation.
- **Do you compare yourself with others too much?** Some candidates seem to delight in upsetting the 'opposition' during revision and exams and it is important to have a positive view of your own abilities. (Expect some degree of hysteria and gamesmanship on revision courses.)
- Do you find it helpful to make your own detailed notes, or do you prefer to highlight important facts in your textbooks?
- Do you **use others to help you learn**? This can help you to practise parts of the exam (like MCQs) and clarify difficult areas as well as offering a useful source of support. Do you work best by yourself, or as part of a group? Many find that a combination of approaches is most effective. Consider meeting once weekly for several hours with other colleagues who are doing the exam. **Study groups** like this may provide support as well as assisting with your revision.

Condensing information

There is a large amount of information to learn, and certainly too much to review it all in the few days leading up to the exam. A number of techniques are available to aid rapid review of key information.

Reducing the quantity of information in books/written materials

- Emphasize key areas of text (with highlighters, underlining etc.).
- Cross irrelevant or unclear material out.
- Add new material to margins.

Making notes

- Write long notes (occupying several sheets of A4) and/or short notes (e.g. key words/bullet points).
- Use notes to replace or supplement books.

Other aids to remembering

- Make lists of key information – this can help you to structure what you learn.
- Consider reinforcing your learning by using MCQs to test your learning.

You may find that your ability to remember clinical topics is enhanced by:

- Learning cases/management based around a clinical structure, e.g. the presenting complaint (PC) or history of the presenting complaint (HPC).
- Imagining or writing down details of a 'typical' case that summarizes all the important principles of assessment or management.
- Remembering a specific patient who encompassed a typical (or atypical) presentation, assessment or clinical management plan.

Another possible approach is the use of Mind Maps ® to summarize and structure your learning (see Appendix 2).

Practice

- For *every* candidate **practice is essential**.
- Familiarity with the clinical exam can only be gained through practice. Be merciless in your pursuit of exam practice. **Take every opportunity you can to practise presenting cases** (onward rounds, in clinics etc.) Ask senior colleagues to listen to your presentations and give feedback. Take what *you* find most useful from different approaches and remember that there is no single right way to present a case.
- These practice sessions should mirror the real exam situation as closely as possible, so that you will have built up your confidence in your abilities before you enter the examination room.
- Make sure that you **do mock clinical exams on each of the main areas** that are likely to arise in the exam: all specialties include a group of disorders that lend themselves well to exams and so come up time and time again.
- **Seek supervised training in interviewing skills**. If you can, watch your presentation on video. This is the most effective way of changing your technique and has the added advantage that the actual exam will probably be no more stressful.
- Obtain a copy of the assessment sheet used by the examiners in your clinical exam and **read the advice the relevant College issues to examiners**. A consultant you know who is, or has been, an examiner may be able to help with this.
- **Practise presenting to peers**, and also watch *them* presenting. Attempt to mark each other's performance. You will gain from seeing how others present their cases and they will also learn from you.
- **Try to do mock exams with examiners with different clinical backgrounds**. If there are any College examiners at the hospital where you work, it would be well worth arranging to carry out at least one exam with them as well. **Be willing to accept their feedback** and suggestions for change. Ultimately,

however, you are seeking to develop a clinical interview and presentation style with which *you* are happy.

Postgraduate exams require a much more organized approach than most undergraduate exams. The following sample questions from previous sittings of the exam will give you an opportunity to practise your technique. We suggest that you find two colleagues who are also approaching the MRCS. Set out a chair for the candidate opposite two chairs for the 'examiners'. Rotate your roles so that you all play both examiner and candidate. Although role-play may seem to be a false situation, it is helpful for you to understand the examiners' perspective: most are happy for you to keep going as long as you are talking sense, and subsequent questions are often based on your answers.

Examples of questions asked in a clinical examination

Physiology:

- Pancreatitis, its systemic effects and mediators
- The role of simvastatin in relation to pancreatic secretions
- The Glasgow coma scale
- Raised intracranial pressure, the signs, causes and treatment
- Fistulas, high and low output, proximal and distal
- Meningococcccal disease
- How anti-diabetes drugs work.

Anatomy:

- The thyroid, on a dissection specimen
- The upper limb, on a dissection specimen
- Lumbar vertebra to identify
- 'Describe the vessels on a large bowel angiogram, then discuss the principles of anastomosis and how to do an angiogram'.

(continued)

(continued from previous page)

Pathology:

- Thyroid malignancy, its diagnosis, investigation and classification
- Tumour markers
- 'Identify the appropriate Duke's stage of a tumour after reading the pathology summary'
- Basic microbiology.

Surgery:

- Compartment syndrome, its assessment and management
- How to perform a laparotomy
- How to perform a Zadek's procedure.

The following chapters will address the best way to present yourself, and the information you will have learnt, in each individual section of the MRCS examinations. Much of the content of this book is based on our experience in these settings. The advice and guidelines have been used by many candidates, who have found them helpful for their examinations.

Key points

- ✔ Passing the exam requires a clear revision strategy.
- ✔ Think about the way you learn – is it as effective as it could be?
- ✔ Learn to condense information.
- ✔ Use your daily work to help you learn.
- ✔ Practice is essential.
- ✔ Be prepared to accept constructive feedback.

MRCS Part I-
the MCQs

The MRCS Part I multiple choice question exam

Introduction

The MRCS Part I consists of multiple choice questions (MCQs). The MCQ paper is the most structured of all the MRCS exams. It aims to test the candidate's factual knowledge quickly and reliably. It is necessary to have a thorough knowledge of the subjects in order to pass. This chapter suggests ways of planning your learning with the MCQ exam in mind and describes methods to improve your MCQ technique so that you are able to use your knowledge more effectively.

It is important to note that the marking scheme used by the different Colleges varies – some (e.g. Edinburgh) use a *negative* marking scheme; others (e.g. Glasgow) use a *neutral* marking scheme. The marking format has important implications for your approach to answering the questions and will be described in detail later in the chapter.

Preparing for the MCQ exam

- Produce a clear revision timetable in order to cover each area adequately. You will need to **start your revision well before the exam** if you are going to cover all the subject areas.
- It is often useful to **go on a course at the very beginning of your revision**. There are several advantages – it can help you get your revision going, boost your motivation, and highlight areas of weakness on which to focus your learning. It also allows you to realize the depth of knowledge that you must aim for and the amount of time you need to set aside for your revision.

- Commercially-run **'crammer' courses** are a valuable way to gain further teaching and practise MCQs under exam conditions. Although relatively expensive, they can be useful before the exams and will also show you that you are not alone.
- The Royal Colleges publish **distance-learning courses** with teaching days at the College (e.g. the STEP course run by the Royal College of Surgeons of England and the SELECT course by the Royal College of Surgeons of Edinburgh). Many candidates undertake these distance-learning packages and the reported pass-rate for these candidates is high.
- You may be fortunate enough to work in a unit or region that runs its own revision course or study days – **take advantage of any local teaching or mock exams**.

MCQ contents

The Colleges all publish a syllabus list – obtain and read it. It will list the areas that the College (and hence the examiners) believes are important. Most of the Colleges separate subjects into 'core' or 'system' sections. These are sometimes arbitrary divisions as many subjects could be included in either.

Core subjects

- Preoperative management
- Anaesthesia
- Intraoperative care
- Postoperative care
- Theatre procedures
- Surgical technique
- Sepsis management
- Trauma/burns
- Critical care/resuscitation
- Neoplasia
- Operative anatomy

System subjects

- Gastrointestinal surgery
- Vascular surgery
- Head and neck surgery
- Orthopaedics
- Urology
- Breast surgery
- Cardiothoracic surgery
- Neurosurgery
- Endocrinology
- Plastic surgery
- Paediatric surgery
- Minimal-access surgery

You must have a good knowledge of the core subjects, but many candidates concentrate so much on these that they pay inadequate attention to the less common topics. Building these into your study plan could give you an advantage.

Time spent on the so-called 'fringe' subjects may also be very productive. The College databases have fewer questions on these topics, they tend to be more straightforward, and are often to be found in the MCQ books.

Fringe subjects

- Audit
- Nutrition
- Sports injuries
- Statistics
- Screening
- Radiotherapy/chemotherapy
- Consent issues

The following topics have also repeatedly been included in Part I and Part II exams.

- Elementary statistics

- Epidemiology
- Clinical sciences
- Basic sciences.

Despite the move away from pure science questions, candidates will still be expected to have sound basic knowledge of anatomy, physiology and pathology. These will often be disguised in a clinical question (e.g. what you know about the relationship of the hypoglossal nerve to the carotid artery may be examined in a question on what nerves may be at risk during carotid endarterectomy).

Other subjects that are less frequently included are:

- Immunology
- Genetics
- Biochemistry
- Microbiology
- Pharmacology
- Principles of cell biology.

Some conditions appear more frequently in MCQ exams than they do in clinical practice and it is worth paying them disproportionate attention. The following list includes some examples.

- HIV and Hepatitis (B and C)
- Sterilization procedures
- Metabolic response to injury
- Coagulopathy
- Sepsis
- Antibiotic prophylaxis.

If you had only 1 hour left before the exam, it would probably be more productive to read notes on several of these topics than on a large subject area such as vascular surgery.

Sources of information

Clearly it would be impossible to obtain an individual textbook on each of these subjects and read it to a depth necessary to answer every multiple choice question. The best way of approaching this problem is therefore to choose a relatively simple system-specific textbook. Read it from cover to cover, trying to understand the basic principles thoroughly. Textbooks that cover the core subjects well include those listed below.

Suitable textbooks for core subjects

General Surgery

- *Bailey and Love's Short Practice of Surgery*[1]
- *Essential Surgery*[2]
- *The New Aird's Companion to Surgical Studies*[3]
- *Surgery* (the journal)[4]

Orthopaedics

- *Textbook of Orthopaedics and Fractures*[5]
- *Louis Apley's System of Orthopaedics and Fractures*[6]
- *Essential Orthopaedics and Trauma*[7]

Critical Care

- *Intensive Care Manual*[8]

MCQs

- *Self-assessment MCQs*[9]
- *MCQs in Applied Basic Science for Basic Surgical Training.*[10]

This list is not exhaustive, but indicates the level of knowledge that you should be seeking to acquire. You will need to supplement this reading with more focused learning from other sources. These should include more specialized textbooks and basic science textbooks. Increasingly, internet sites are becoming a valuable resource for MCQ questions, e.g. *www.surgical-tutor.org.uk*

You must make sure that you feel comfortable with the style and 'readability' of your main book as it is likely that you will end up reading large parts of it several times. It is often better to start with smaller, more manageable books (these may include textbooks that you have used as an undergraduate). The advantages of using these books is that most of the basic knowledge will be familiar and can be covered fairly quickly. Completing the book may give you a sense of satisfaction at having accomplished some revision in a short period, rather than that feeling of endless ploughing through a large volume.

Examples of smaller more manageable texts

- The 'ABC' books published by the BMJ Publishing Group (e.g. *Breast Diseases, Colorectal Diseases, Major Trauma, Nutrition, Sports Medicine, Transfusion, Urology, Vascular Diseases*)
- *Surgical Diagnosis and Management*[11]

The Royal College of Surgeons Course Manual, *Clinical Surgery in General*[12], is a useful text which addresses the smaller topics as well as the more conventional areas of surgery.

Know when to stop buying/reading new material

One danger to avoid is thinking that you *must* read *everything*. There are almost unlimited numbers of books and papers that you could read. Because of this, you need to define your learning boundaries clearly: as well as deciding what materials to use for your revision, part of prioritizing your learning is to decide what *not* to use. A time must come in every revision plan when it is more helpful to concentrate on re-revising material you have already learnt. When you reach this point, make a conscious decision not to buy or borrow any more books and, instead, focus on learning what you have already read more effectively.

Using MCQs to help you revise

At the beginning of your preparation for the exam **it is useful to spend some time *writing* MCQs**. For example, after completing a chapter of a book, try to write a few MCQs on the subject you have just learned. This helps to test and reinforce your knowledge and will highlight the kind of information that is amenable to multiple choice questioning. The questions are also useful for later revision. As you read through your textbooks, mark facts which are 'MCQ-able' with a highlighter pen. The number of straightforward true/false facts is actually remarkably small. This will help you focus your learning.

Using MCQ questions to help you learn

A few MCQ books for surgery are available. Some of these are better (and more accurate) than others. Some books contain whole papers of mixed questions; others consist of questions organized by topic. The most useful multiple choice questions are those published by the Colleges, as these are written by the College examiners.

- Make sure that you attempt some of the College MCQs at the start of your revision – this will set a standard to revise towards.
- **Make your revision more interesting by using MCQs.** Some people find that when they continually revise a set of notes over a period of weeks they cease to take in any new information. One way of preventing this is to practise MCQs on each topic shortly after you have revised it.
- MCQ books can help identify the sort of information which is asked in MCQ exams. **Improve your factual knowledge base by testing yourself with MCQs.** If you find you do badly in a particular topic, target your reading towards this area, looking for the answers to the questions that you got wrong. This helps to highlight the areas of a subject which are important, and allows you to augment or improve your notes.
- Do not try to remember hundreds of dislocated facts. Instead, try to **integrate information you learn with your existing knowledge** so that you understand the principles involved. Summary notes may help you do this. Of most value are books which explain the answers so that you add to your knowledge.

Subject spotting

Exam courses often emphasize 'subject spotting'. They suggest that, by analysing previous papers and measuring the frequency of questions on different subjects, it is possible to target revision at specific exam-orientated subjects. This is of limited value, however, as the content of different exams varies significantly. What *is* important to remember is that you *must* know and understand the core and system subjects well.

MCQ technique

Some Colleges use *negative* marking for MCQ papers and others use a *neutral* system. It is important to understand the different techniques needed to answer each type of MCQ.

What is the difference between neutral and negative marking?

In **neutral marking** a mark is gained for every correct response you make. *No* marks are awarded for an incorrect response or for a question that is left blank. The implication of this is that **you should attempt to answer every question** in a neutrally-marked exam as there is no penalty for an incorrect response. For example, if in the exam there are 20 MCQ questions for which you cannot think of the correct answer, you *should* make a response to them, as even complete guesses are likely to gain a 50% mark and an average of 10 points (if the number of true and false answers in the paper are evenly distributed).

In **negative marking** a mark will be awarded for each correct answer, no marks for a 'don't know' response, and one mark will be *deducted* for an incorrect response. The implication of this is that you need to be fairly confident in your answers as each incorrect response will lose you a mark. For example, if you answer all the questions of a paper, and score 70% right and 30% wrong your net score would be only 40%. Even very knowledgeable candidates can fail exams marked this way as a result of poor exam technique. In negatively-marked papers, choosing *not* to attempt questions for which you have no idea of the answer can be a useful strategy.

Scores in neutrally-marked and negatively-marked papers:

Answer	Neutrally-marked examination	Negatively-marked examination
Correct answer	+1	+1
'Don't know' or blank response	0	0
Wrong response	0	−1

Basic MCQ techniques

- **Read the whole question very carefully** and break it down into individual facts. Mark each of these facts as true or false. Read each stem and item as a single sentence.
- Be particularly careful with questions on the topics which you feel confident about. Your elation may lead you to misread the question and lose marks where you should have gained them. (A colleague of ours had made a particular point of learning the anatomical relations of the ureter. He was therefore delighted to find this exact question in an exam paper. Unfortunately he gained no marks because the question was about the anatomical relations of the *urethra*.)
- Have you understood the question? Beware of double negatives – one in the question and one in the stem. Examiners do try to avoid setting such questions but they crop up occasionally.
- Make sure you **put each answer onto the right line of the answer sheet** and check this frequently. It is easy to get your answers out of order. This will cause panic and could cost you the exam. Build in a review every ten minutes or so to make sure that the correct answer is still being placed on the correct line of the paper. It is a disaster to notice two minutes

before the end of the exam that you have transcribed the questions onto the answer sheet incorrectly.

- **Review your progress regularly** to make sure that you will complete the paper.
- Ruthlessly **skip those questions where you really don't know the answer and come back to them later**. You may find that other questions trigger your memory and the answer comes to you later in the exam.

Don't be *too* clever

Don't be too clever and automatically assume that the examiners are trying to trick you. **Avoid agonizing over possible hidden meanings**, as this is more likely to hinder rather than help your decisions. **In MCQs, the 'correct' answer to a question is the generally accepted version of the truth**. If you have some special knowledge of a topic that is at variance with the most prevalent viewpoint – swallow your pride and save it for the viva!

Example 1

The following facts about our solar system are true:

a) It takes 365 days for the Earth to orbit the Sun
b) The same side of the Moon is always visible from the Earth
c) The Moon circles the Earth every 28 days
d) Gravity is related to the speed of rotation of a planet
e) Only planets with an iron core have a magnetic field.

- The answer to stem **a)** is true. However, the very knowledgeable candidate may be aware that the Earth takes *365.27* days to circulate the Sun and he or she may then answer this as false. The number given, 365, is 'near enough' right.
- The same side of the Moon *is* always visible from Earth and therefore stem **b)** is true. However, there is a phenomenon called 'libration', a consequence of

---

(continued)

(continued from previous page)

which is that 59% of the Moon's surface is visible, but at different times. If the candidate is aware of this he or she may then answer this question incorrectly as false. This is reading too much into the question.

- The answer to stem **c)** is true. However, once again, the very knowledgeable candidate may be aware that the Moon takes *27.3* days to circulate the Earth and he or she may then answer this as false. This is being too precise. The answer, 28 days, is near enough.
- The answer to stem **d)** is false. Gravity is related to the mass of an object. This is a question you can only answer if you have specific knowledge about this fact.
- Categorical words such as 'only' and 'always' and 'never' often indicate that the answer is false. It is very rare for a finding to apply in only *one* situation. The answer to stem **e)** is therefore likely to be (and in fact *is*) false.

It is also possible to be too clever by adding to the information that you have been given. With a little bit of ingenuity and lateral thinking, it is possible to make *almost anything* true. **Answer the question, simply, as it is written**.

Example 2

An elevated blood sugar is a recognized feature of ulcerative colitis – true or false?

- This is false but as many patients with ulcerative colitis will be on steroids which can precipitate a high blood sugar in certain individuals, some candidates may mark the question true.

Extended Matching MCQs

'Extended matching' questions are used in the MRCS MCQs. They are less common than 'normal format' questions but still comprise a significant percentage of the questions. **They are used to assess the use of *reasoning* to answer questions** not just the simple regurgitation of facts.

Each question has a theme (e.g. thyroid disease). Several diagnostic options are available, related to the main heading. The question usually describes a case scenario and the candidate is asked to match this with the most likely diagnosis from the list of options. Each case presented will have only *one* correct answer from the list.

Example 1

Thyroid disease

a) Thyroglossal duct cyst
b) Thyrotoxicosis
c) Ectopic thyroid
d) Multinodular colloid goitre
e) Anaplastic carcinoma
f) Papillary carcinoma

For each of the patients described below choose the most likely diagnosis from the options above.

Question 1: An 8-year-old girl is referred to a paediatrician with a slow-growing, non-tender, firm thyroid lump and non-tender cervical lymphadenopathy. **Answer – f)**

Question 2: A 19-year-old man with a non-tender, midline, anterior cervical swelling which moves on swallowing and protrusion of the tongue. **Answer – a)**

Question 3: A 45-year-old woman presents to her GP with weight loss, diarrhoea, an irregular pulse and insomnia. **Answer – b)**

Core subjects will also be presented in an extended matching format.

Example 2

Suture materials

a) Polyglactin
b) Stainless steel wire
c) PDS
d) Catgut
e) Polypropylene
f) Silk

Question 1: A synthetic non-absorbable polymer, used as a monofilament suture. Popular for skin closure. **Answer – e)**

Question 2: A synthetic, braided, absorbable suture, it causes minimal tissue reaction. Absorbed in 60–90 days. **Answer – a)**

Question 3: A synthetic monofilament absorbable suture, absorbed by tissue hydrolysis, causes minimal tissue reaction. Completely absorbed in 180 days. **Answer – c)**

Do not try to 'fool the system' by putting more than one answer for each question – if this happens the question will be discounted automatically. Occasionally, one answer from the list is the correct one for more than one of the questions: do not let this put you off from using it as an answer. By approaching each part of the question logically, a good attempt can be made at answering. There are several new textbooks that provide practice in extended matching questions.[13,14]

Be aware of the techniques examiners use in writing questions

It is surprisingly difficult to write good MCQs. Understanding some of the techniques used by examiners in writing questions will help you to avoid some of the possible pitfalls. It is useful to think about questions from the perspective of the person writing them. They will wish to have a spread of true and false responses, of varying degrees of difficulty. Ideally, the questions will enable them to discriminate between those who know a subject well and those whose knowledge is superficial. Unfortunately for you, the techniques used to construct questions may mean that a *little* knowledge can make it more likely that the incorrect answer is chosen – this is particularly true when the correct answer is 'false'.

It is relatively easy to formulate 'true' questions. Read a chapter in a textbook and see how easy it is to pick out five facts that are true. The question can be made more difficult either by choosing obscure facts or by expressing the question in a form that is unlikely to have been read in a textbook, but can be worked out if the subject is known well. It is possible that you will sometimes know the answer to a question but not realize it. This is because the question has been **phrased in an unexpected way** or because it occurs in an unexpected place.

Example

In a patient with Crohn's disease:

a) Urinary oxalate concentration may be elevated.

In your reading about Crohn's disease you will probably *not* have read that urinary oxalate concentration can be elevated. However, you would probably be aware that up to one-fifth of Crohn's patients will develop renal calculi and more specifically, oxalate stones. Therefore, you should be able to work out that the answer is 'true' even if you initially thought you did not know the answer.

Overall, you should be confident about your 'true' answers – after all, you are answering it as 'true' because you have seen or heard it somewhere before. **It is much more difficult to be confident about your 'false' answers** – the fact that you think that 'A is not a feature of B' may simply reflect that you do not know much about the subject! When a negative-marking scheme is used, this can sometimes cause problems when a candidate has a feeling (but does not know for sure) that a response is incorrect. You will find out more about how to approach this situation later.

It is much more difficult for the examiners to write good 'false' questions. These may be created by using popular misconceptions or by using the *opposite* of the truth. **Candidates are more likely not to answer a question if the correct answer is 'false'** rather than if it is 'true'. Therefore, being able to answer the 'false' questions correctly can give you an edge over other candidates, and can be a very valuable source of extra marks. In order to answer a question as 'false' you need to have an extensive knowledge of the subject. You need to be more careful when answering 'false' rather than 'true', except when you recognize that a 'switch' has occurred and you know confidently that the opposite is true.

Recognizing a 'switch'
The following can be switched:

- nouns (or diseases)
- adjectives
- negative to positive, or vice versa.

Example 1

The following statements are true about the planets:

a) Jupiter has a great dark spot
b) The hottest planet is Mercury.

The answer to stem **a)** is false. If the candidate remembers that Jupiter has a spot he may well answer this as true; unfortunately for him, Jupiter has a *red* spot (Neptune has a dark spot). **This stem has been created by switching words or by mixing known facts**. Here a little knowledge is likely to make an 'educated' guess wrong.

The answer to stem **b)** is false. If the candidate knows that Mercury is the nearest planet to the Sun she may answer this question as true. Venus, the second-nearest planet to the Sun, is the hottest planet, however, as it

---

(continued)

41

(continued from previous page)

possesses an atmosphere and is affected by the greenhouse effect. **This question has been created by switching key words**.

Example 2

In a patient with gallstones:

a) Cholesterol stones are commonly radio-opaque
b) There is an association with ulcerative colitis
c) Large bowel obstruction is a recognized complication
d) Unconjugated hyperbilirubinaemia occurs if a stone obstructs the common bile duct
e) Cholecystitis can lead to gram-positive septicaemic shock.

If a candidate knows that:

- *Some* gallstones can be radio-opaque (pigment stones)
- Gallstones can be associated with *inflammatory bowel disease* (*Crohn's*)
- *Small* bowel obstruction can complicate gallstones (gallstone ileus)
- *Conjugated* hyperbilirubinaemia occurs if a stone obstructs the common bile duct
- Cholecystitis can lead to *gram-negative* septicaemic shock

. . . it is possible that he or she may make a calculated guess that the above statements are all true. In fact they are all false. **The questions have been constructed by taking a known fact and exchanging a key word**. It is important that candidates are aware of this technique for writing questions and the pitfalls it may cause.

Example 3

The following statements are true in splenectomy:

a) Overwhelming post-splenectomy sepsis occurs in 15% of cases
b) Immunoglobulin-M levels rise following splenectomy
c) There is considerable intersegmental arterial blood flow
d) Pneumococcal vaccine in elective patients should preferably be given 2 weeks postoperatively
e) Post-splenectomy, the platelet count reaches its lowest level after 7–10 days.

All of these answers are false. **The question has been created by reading a textbook, picking out facts and 'switching' the correct answer**. If they are recognized as a switch they can be answered as false.

Example 4

Pancreatitis can be precipitated by a low plasma calcium concentration.

You know, or should do, that pancreatitis is associated with a *high* plasma calcium concentration and it is therefore easy to recognize that the opposite is true and that this answer is therefore false.

The wording of the question

It is important to look at questions from two perspectives: factual knowledge and logic. If the questions are well written it should be impossible to answer them without any knowledge of the subject. However, good MCQs are difficult to write and many questions contain some clues within the structure of the question. Use your common sense.

Three particularly common stems are:

- A '**characteristic feature**' means that it is of diagnostic significance. Its absence might make one doubt the diagnosis. If it is truly characteristic then you are likely to be aware of it.
- A '**typical feature**' is one that you would expect to be present. It is similar to 'characteristic'.
- A '**recognized feature**' is one that, although it may not *characterize* a disease, has been reported. Marking this as false implies an in-depth knowledge of the subject, unless it can be recognized as a switch.

Other terminology

- ' . . . **is a pathognomonic feature**' means that it occurs only in that condition. If you do not know the answer then it is likely to be false. There are few pathognomonic features and you are likely to know them.
- ' . . . **is associated with**' means that it is a feature which is well recognized but not common. The same applies to ' . . . **is a recognized feature of**'.
- Categorical statements including words such as '**never**', '**always**', '**only**', or '**invariably**' should be answered as *false*, unless you are *sure* that they are true.
- Statements containing words such as '**possible**', '**may**', '**rarely**' or '**can**' tend to be *true*.

The exam paper may include precise definitions of phrases such as 'pathognomonic', so **read the introduction to the paper carefully** rather than diving into the questions. The definitions may alter the answer you choose significantly.

Use your sense of logic
The following techniques may help you clarify your thinking about an answer:

- Look for terminology that is likely to make a question true or false
- Reversing the question (e.g. 'X *may not* occur in Y') can help clarify your thinking. Try this with some questions in any MCQ book to illustrate how helpful this technique is.

> **Example 1**
>
> *In phaeochromocytoma*:
>
> *a) There is unlikely to be a family history of the disease.*
>
> Reversing the question leads to 'In phaeochromocytoma there may be a family history . . . '. This would make it more likely that you would give the correct answer which is 'true'.

Look for items that are **contradictory**. Contradictory items should not be included within one question as they would be immediately obvious. However, they may be included in different questions in the same paper and this can offer you additional clues.

> **Example 2**
>
> *In ketoacidosis*:
>
> a) The pH is likely to be low (True)
> b) The hydrogen ion concentration is likely to be low (False)
> c) There is a decrease in organic acids (False)
>
> Clearly, *all* of these items cannot be true.
>
> - The answers to a) and b) *cannot* be the same.
> - The answers to a) and c) are *unlikely* to be the same.

Advanced MCQ technique for negatively-marked papers

This section is only relevant for *negatively*-marked exams. If you are sitting a *neutrally*-marked exam, skip straight to *Timing and practical issues*.

Testing your 'feeling of knowing'

In a negatively-marked exam, one mark will be awarded for each correct answer, *no* marks will be awarded for a 'don't know' response, and one mark will be *deducted* for an incorrect response. This marking approach was introduced in order to discourage candidates from guessing. In theory, if you haven't a clue about the answer, a complete guess should have an equal chance of being correct or incorrect, resulting in an average score of zero marks. In practice however, some people seem to be naturally better at answering MCQ questions than others and will score highly because of their ability to make a confident, calculated guess. This *'feeling of knowing'* that candidates experience when they read certain questions has been researched. When you do an MCQ paper, you will find that you:

- *Know* the answer with a high degree of certainty
- Definitely know that you *don't know* the answer
- Have a *'feeling of knowing'* that the answer is correct, but are *not quite* sure.

Studies show that the accuracy of people's 'feeling of knowing' varies. Even allowing for negative marking, most people will finish up with a net positive mark if they act in response to their 'gut feelings' concerning the right answer. It is important to know if this general statistical finding is true for you. It is our experience that **approximately one in eight candidates are not able to trust their 'feeling of knowing'**: for whatever reason, if they trust their gut feeling, they will be more often wrong than right. **This can have disastrous results in a negatively-marked exam**. If you have found that throughout your exam career you have persistently experienced problems passing negatively-marked MCQs, you may be one of these people. You need to find out if you are because this has important implications for how you should approach the exam.

To find this out, do several MCQ papers covering a range of topics. As you do each paper, mark your answers using either a black or a red pen:

- If you know the answer, mark it in *black*
- If you don't know the answer, leave it *blank*
- If you have a 'feeling of knowing' mark it in *red*.

Now go through the papers and mark them: compare your score when you were certain with any additional marks you would have gained using your 'feeling of knowing'. If you find that over a series of papers you have made a net gain of marks by using your instincts, keep doing it. If not, then be cautious about answering questions on a negatively-marked paper unless you are at least *reasonably* sure about the answer.

The confidence test

Consider carrying out a more detailed analysis on your answers on several MCQ papers. Try to identify if there are areas of knowledge in which you have a particularly low level or high level of knowledge (e.g. you may have a greater confidence in general surgery than in endocrine surgery). If you find that many of your 'certain' answers are wrong, you may be *overconfident* about your knowledge and need to do more factual revision.

There are some people whose inner doubts prevent them from making 'false' responses to questions that they think are incorrect. As a result, they tend to answer such questions too often as 'don't know'. To test yourself, complete several MCQ papers using your normal answering style. Repeat the papers after changing your strategy by answering more questions which you think are wrong as false. Compare your marks using this strategy with your usual answering style. Do you gain or lose marks using this technique? If you are consistently gaining marks, you should actively consider altering your threshold of response.

Timing and practical issues

Check the up-to-date College examination instructions and regulations to find out how many questions you have to complete and what time is allocated – the structure and content of the exams may change. There is usually more than enough time to complete the paper. You should allow some time at the end to check your answers, especially if you have marked the answers on the question sheet before transferring them to the answer sheet. You must be strict with timing and work out in advance the time that you will allocate to each block of questions. Don't waste time at the end counting your answers – answer as many as you can.

Finally, if you are finding the paper extremely difficult, it is likely that others are too. **Do not give up**. Carry on and try to finish. Do not leave the exam hall in despair – you *can* still pass.

Using these techniques may help you gain some extra marks, but **there is no substitute for developing broad-based knowledge**. Practise answering as many MCQs as possible, giving consideration to the *style* of question as well as the factual answer.

Key points

- ✔ Make sure you know the structure of the exam.
- ✔ Start your revision early.
- ✔ Concentrate initially on obtaining a solid understanding of the subject matter.
- ✔ Practise using a variety of MCQ books and use MCQs to help you revise.
- ✔ Start concentrating on MCQ-able facts at least 6–8 weeks before the exam.
- ✔ Work to perfect your technique.
- ✔ Don't panic: exam papers often seem very difficult. Do not leave the exam because of fears that you are doing badly: it is likely that everyone else is finding it hard too.
- ✔ Read the questions very carefully and look for clues in the wording.
- ✔ Keep checking that your answers are in the correct place on the answer sheet.

(continued)

(continued from previous page)

> ✔ Maintain momentum.
>
> On a *negatively*-marked exam:
>
> ✔ Test whether you can trust your 'feeling of knowing'.
> ✔ Complete a confidence analysis – the 'don't know' test.
>
> On a *neutrally*-marked exam:
>
> ✔ Answer *all* the questions – don't leave any blank.

Acknowledgements
This chapter is based on a chapter written by Chris Williams, David Protheroe and Keith Brownlee in *Pass the MRCPsych*, Second edition. WB Saunders: Edinburgh (2000).

REFERENCES

1). Russell RCG, Williams NS, Bulstrode CJK (2000) *Bailey and Love's Short Practice of Surgery*, 23rd edn. Arnold: London.

2). Burkitt HG, Quick CRG, Deakin PJ (2001) *Essential Surgery*, 3rd edn. Churchill Livingstone: Edinburgh.

3). Burnand KG, Young AE (1998) *The New Aird's Companion to Surgical Studies*, 2nd edn. Churchill Livingstone: Edinburgh.

4). *Surgery*. The Medicine Publishing Group: Abingdon.

5). Hughes SPF, Porter RW (1997) *Textbook of Orthopaedics and Fractures*. Arnold: London.

6). Apley AG (1993) *Louis Apley's System of Orthopaedics and Fractures*, 7th edn. Butterworth Heinmann: Oxford.

7). Dandy DJ (1998) *Essential Orthopaedics and Trauma*, 3rd edn. Churchill Livingstone: Edinburgh.

8). Oh TE (1996) *Intensive Care Manual*, 4th edn. Butterworth Heinmann: Oxford.

9). *Self-assessment MCQs.* (1997) The Royal College of Surgeons of Edinburgh, Nicolson Street, Edinburgh, EH8 9DW, UK. Tel: 0131 527 1600.

10). Jacob S (2000) *MCQs in Applied Basic Science for Basic Surgical Training.* Churchill Livingstone: Edinburgh.

11). Dunn DC (1999) *Surgical Diagnosis and Management,* 3rd edn. Blackwell Science: Oxford.

12). Kirk RM (1999) *Clinical Surgery in General* (Royal College of Surgeons Course Manual) 3rd edn. Churchill Livingstone: Edinburgh.

13). Chatrath P, Rahim O (1999) *MRCS examination: MCQs and EMQs.* Blackwell Science: Oxford.

14). Williams A (1998) *MRCS core modules: MCQs and EMQs.* PasTest.

FURTHER READING

15). Huang JKC, Winslet MC (2000) *The Complete MRCS: Volume I Core Modules.* Churchill Livingstone: Edinburgh.

16). Huang JKC, Winslet MC (2000) *The Complete MRCS: Volume 2 System Modules.* Churchill Livingstone: Edinburgh.

MRCS Part II-
the clinicals

Revision strategy for the clinical examinations

Thorough preparation for the clinical exam is essential but often neglected. You would not dream of preparing for your driving test only by reading the *Highway Code* and not practising your driving. The clinical exam is totally different from the MCQ: not only are you required to have an excellent factual knowledge, you must be able to apply it clinically. Spend time learning how to present your answers effectively.

It will be necessary to demonstrate the skills required in taking a concise history and examining a patient, as well as the communication skills needed to present the case to the examiners and the factual knowledge to enable you to answer questions on your findings.

How to prepare

Regular practice at short cases will significantly improve your ability to take a structured and directed history, examine a patient systematically, and present a clear summary to an examiner.

It is very difficult to prepare adequately for the clinical exam completely by yourself. **Consider working with a group of candidates who are applying for the same exam**. Organize teaching opportunities for the entire group, enlisting the help of cooperative patients, especially those who have interesting symptoms or clinical signs. Studying as part of a group enables you to compare your level of knowledge with that of your peers and provides valuable experience in performing clinical examination in front of others. **The more clinical teaching you receive the better**. Take every opportunity to practise presenting and answering questions.

Use your job to help you revise. Treat every patient that you see in accident and emergency and outpatients as a potential exam case: try not to read the general practitioner's referral letter first but approach the case afresh; if asked to see someone with abdominal pain, assess the patient *before* looking at the blood results; if asked to see someone with a fracture of the neck of femur, examine the patient *before* looking at the X-ray. Always take a good social history and think through how your patient's illness will affect them.

Factual knowledge required

During your revision you should be developing:

- Knowledge
- Judgement
- Precision in answering questions.

You may be presented with:

- Cases from everyday practice
- Rare disorders
- Unusual manifestations of common conditions.

Ideally you should have an in-depth knowledge of the standard recommended surgical textbooks, supplemented by further reading from specialist books and journals. Do not despair – it is clearly impossible to learn *all* the available material. It is a popular misconception that you need to know all about everything.

You should aim to have a working knowledge across all the main surgical specialties as a basic foundation of knowledge, and should supplement this with more detailed study in the smaller specialties.

Read one of the undergraduate surgical textbooks from cover to cover and know it back to front, as candidates often fail through not knowing common topics well, rather than not knowing the rare conditions. You will find it relatively easy and it will give you a broad knowledge base. The *Surgery* journal series and the College distance-learning courses are also useful and have the advantage of being regularly updated.

Spread your learning effectively. Your more detailed study should span as many specialties as possible. Remember that it is an exam which tests the *breadth* of your surgical knowledge. You should avoid getting bogged down trying to learn one or two subjects in very great detail while completely neglecting other areas of surgery. While you might wish to become a great authority on the minutiae of, for instance, thyroid surgery this will not help you with most of the questions. **Broadly speaking, you should cover the same specialties as were recommended for Part I of the exam**.

One important danger to avoid is thinking that you must read *everything*. There is an almost unlimited number of books and papers you could read. Part of prioritizing your learning is to decide what materials *not* to learn from: a time comes in everyone's revision when it is more helpful to concentrate on re-revising materials that have already been learnt.

Using sample questions

Ask your colleagues who have already sat the exam for a list of the questions they encountered. This will help you to familiarize yourself with the focus and standard of the questions that are asked. The sooner this is done after the exam, the better their recall will be.

Use of exam practice books

One way of maintaining variety and of keeping your study broadly based is to use the books that concentrate on questions, data interpretation and photographic material which are aimed specifically at candidates sitting the MRCS examination. There are an increasing number of books addressing the short cases and viva techniques. FRCS books can also be used as revision for the MRCS exams, particularly the viva revision texts.

These texts have the advantage that they will familiarize you with some of the rare conditions you may come across in the exam and are a welcome diversion from struggling through textbooks. That having been said, however, exam-orientated books can be used to stimulate more detailed reading in larger general or specialist textbooks, and help you to focus your learning on areas that commonly come up in the exam. It is a mistake to rely exclusively on these specialist membership books or upon books of lists. **You will have a greater chance of getting the right answer by *understanding* subjects rather than by learning facts by rote.**

Exam strategy

The membership exam is not just about learning facts, but also about how you use your knowledge effectively as a good clinician. Many candidates expect the exam to be a straightforward regurgitation of factual knowledge in the form of a list. They are surprised how difficult it is to answer the questions fully, even when the question is about a topic with which they feel very familiar. As in clinical practice, there may be a number of correct answers, but you may be asked for only one. In other words, your judgement will also be tested: **it is**

important that you develop the skill of selecting the *most likely* from a list of possibilities. For instance you may know a long list of causes of hepatosplenomegaly, but not be able to select the one that most closely fits the information you have been given.

The examiner does not make a decision as to whether each of the questions is 'passed' or 'failed'. You can get a rare diagnosis wrong but still score marks for suggesting appropriate investigations. Marks are awarded in a predetermined manner and **very specific answers are often required**. Vague, incomplete or partly wrong answers will score low or no marks. It is possible to know the correct answer, but fail to get the maximum number of available marks because you were not sufficiently precise. For instance, if given some arterial blood gases to interpret, 'metabolic acidosis' would score more marks than 'acidosis'. If shown a photograph of an X-ray and the correct answer is 'left pneumothorax' the candidate would probably only get half-marks (or would at least lose some marks) if they only answer 'pneumothorax'.

To do well in the clinical exams you must *organize* your knowledge, making sure that what you say is:

- Clear
- Relevant
- Interesting.

Remember that the purpose of the exam is to identify a safe, competent and professional practitioner. It is more important to have a solid grasp of the basic principles of treatment than of the fine detail. Previous candidates will claim that they failed for all sorts of trivial reasons. One candidate claimed that he failed because he did not know any of the causative organisms of mycotic aneurysms. Rumours like this appear frequently and may be spread by unsuccessful previous candidates. Do not allow them to reduce your confidence or commitment to pass.

> ### Key points
>
> ✔ There is no substitute for broad-based knowledge and understanding.
> ✔ Use every opportunity in your clinical work to practise systematic examination and presentation.
> ✔ Consider *all* the information you have been given.
> ✔ Develop the skill of weighing-up the significance of different 'right' answers.
> ✔ Answer as precisely and concisely as you can.
>
> ### Remember
>
> ✔ You have done this before.
> ✔ Clear communicators consistently do well in the clinical.
> ✔ You are presenting *yourself,* not merely the case.
> ✔ You are being asked to demonstrate your skills as a safe, competent clinician.

Going to the exam

Before the exam

Before you set out for the exam, you need to consider carefully some practical issues that may make or break your overall presentation:

- What will I wear?
- What impression do I want to give (– clothes, haircut etc.)?
- What will I do over the lunchtime break? (Do not come back smelling of drink, smoke, garlic or curry!)

How can I arrive on time?

It is surprising how often this causes problems: expect the unexpected (traffic jams, rail strikes, losing your car keys, etc.). If you are late for any part of the exam it is likely that this will leave you feeling tense and pressured and unlikely to perform as well as you would if you were not so flustered. Being late can destroy months of hard work and means that you will have to repeat all your revision if you fail. Definitely consider staying overnight in a 'nice' quiet hotel – it is worth the money. Some hotels offer reduced rates for MRCS candidates; others may offer corporate rates for your hospital Trust. A long drive, with an early start, can seem too far on the actual day and will leave you feeling stressed. You will probably not have slept well either. If, when you book into your hotel, you find that it is being renovated or is dirty or noisy, consider leaving. The cost of a hotel bill is insignificant when compared with the personal cost of failing the exam simply because you had a sleepless night because of a hotel party.

The exam itself

It is essential to arrive in plenty of time for everything. Before examining a patient always listen to any comments made by the examiners. Try to maintain a calm outward appearance even if it feels as though your brain is in turmoil. The examiners will allow you a few seconds to consider your answer and a short silence appears more professional than a panicky answer.

Some abbreviations are so universally used that they are acceptable answers. 'ECG' and 'CT' are possible examples of this type, but if you are in any doubt it is worth using the full name. Other, less universal abbreviations are not safe to use. For example, 'TOF' could be taken to mean either tracheo-oesophageal fistula or Tetralogy of Fallot.

A few of the questions will seem especially difficult. You may find that you are not sure what the examiner is asking for and so do not feel able to proceed with an answer. Do not panic. Ask the examiner to rephrase the question. Remember that any question that seems very hard for you is probably also very hard for everyone else. However, don't do this *too* often, as it will look like time-wasting.

Try to imagine you are encountering this problem in everyday clinical practice, for example in accident and emergency or in outpatients. Decide what you would do in clinical practice. Try to forget that you are in an exam.

The best environment to learn this is therefore a busy surgical job in the relevant specialties. No amount of book reading will make up for a deficit in clinical awareness and the skills gained in the day-to-day practice of surgery. During your senior house officer years, you should learn from your seniors (including radiologists and other specialists) and take every opportunity to discuss the reasoning behind the investigation and management of the patients under your care. Merely carrying out a list of duties each day can be both unrewarding and uneducational. Each new patient can be approached as a practice exam case and you should make it the norm to commit yourself to a differential diagnosis, investigation plan and management strategy for every one. Only by doing this regularly will you improve your examination performance and, more importantly, your clinical practice.

The exam aims to test your abilities as an effective and competent clinician. The examiners' key question is 'Would we be happy with you as our specialist registrar?' You need to convey an impression of reliability and safety. In the same way that in a driving test you need to make the instructor feel safe while you drive, **you need to show the examiners that you are a safe, sensible, competent and professional clinician who could be trusted to look after their patients**.

The following chapters go through each aspect of the clinical exams. Do not try to learn the suggestions off by heart. Instead, integrate those areas that you find most helpful into your current approach. **Never change your style of presenting on the day**. You must seek to adopt an approach to the exams which is well learned and practised. Adapt the techniques for yourself, and seek honest (and constructive) feedback from others.

Key points

- ✔ Arrive early. Consider staying in a quiet hotel close to the exam venue.
- ✔ Look smart and professional.
- ✔ You are presenting *yourself*, not just the case.
- ✔ Do not try to change your presentation techniques radically on the day.

6

The short cases

Introduction

For many candidates the short cases are seen as the most difficult hurdle. Even those with good clinical skills and knowledge may experience difficulty with this part of the exam. Preparation is vital, particularly practice under examination conditions. The short cases test your breadth of knowledge and your ability to jump from one system to the next as you would have to in the accident and emergency department, where one moment you may be dealing with pancreatitis and the next with an ischaemic leg. They can involve anything from an end-of-the-bed spot diagnosis, to a full neurological examination or an assessment of knee stability. These are all within the capability of most doctors sitting the MRCS examination, but the key is to be able to perform them whilst under pressure, in the presence of the examiners – and to look as if you have done it a thousand times before. The exam is not the place to do this for the first time. **Your technique must be second nature**: the examination must flow naturally and briskly, and be thorough. This leaves your mind clear to concentrate on your findings and differential diagnosis. Being able to think while you present will mean that you can look for the confirmatory signs or associated findings that will put you one step ahead.

Short case practice

Each new patient you see is an opportunity to practise. This will improve your technique and refine your clinical skills: it will only look like second nature when it *is* second nature.

Try and identify your clinical and academic 'blindspots'. Each of us has areas of knowledge or clinical skills that are less strong than others. Try to identify these and work at improving them to at least a reasonable level.

Practise presenting cases

- **Seek out opportunities to present cases at staff rounds or meetings**: this will give you practice at answering unexpected questions under pressure.
- Seek supervised training in presentation skills. **Watch yourself presenting on video** if possible. This is the most effective way of changing your technique and has the added advantage that the actual exam is likely to be no more stressful in comparison.
- **Arrange a regular session with colleagues who are also sitting the exam** and introduce each other to the exam-orientated cases you have on your wards.
- Find as many 'friendly' specialist registrars as you can and seek regular exam practice with them. It is best to spread the load out between them: producing a printed timetable can help.
- Limit the number of participants at teaching sessions to avoid creating an unmanageable and intimidating group.

Practice sessions provide opportunities for fine-tuning your examination technique. Short, sharp questioning should help you answer under pressure and scrutiny. Remember that you need to be able to substantiate your findings and differential diagnosis.

If you work in a very specialized area, you must make sure that you obtain experience with a wide range of general cases. The reverse is true: it can be helpful to see cases who are being cared for by specialist teams. Obtain varied experience and clinical training in the jobs you choose. Familiarize yourself with local accents and dialects, particularly if English is not your first language.

'Predicting' cases

Try to remember that the hospital where you sit the examination will tend to have the same types of patients that you see in your own clinical practice. The hospital has to provide approximately 50 patients for the short cases and these are therefore likely to include both inpatients and outpatients. Many candidates find it useful to write down full assessment and management plans of a 'typical' case. However, **do not just regurgitate prepared lists** in the exam – remember that every patient is an individual and each case is different. Do not be put off if your findings do not quite 'fit' or are not 'typical': **common conditions may have atypical features**.

If you think that this technique would be useful for you, practise by writing out full assessment and management plans for each of the following and be able to present them concisely and efficiently:

- Ulnar nerve palsy
- Thyroid lump
- Pigmented skin lesion
- Any area that the examining hospital is known to specialize in.

Make sure that you know about current controversies (e.g. laparoscopic colonic resection for malignancy), the names of the common incisions/scars and eponymous names for signs (e.g. Rovsing's, Murphy's, Courvoisier's).

Mock exams

In addition to learning through your general clinical work, you should also seek specific experience in all parts of the exam. Ask your seniors, and especially your consultants, if you can present cases to them on a more formal basis. Most of them will oblige if asked at the correct moment. If there are any Part II clinical examiners at your hospital, try to arrange a mock clinical with them. Be willing to accept their feedback and suggestions for change.

It is best to gain experience in being examined by a range of different people who have different personal styles of examining. Do not omit to practise with examiners who are regarded as 'hard'. This can be an invaluable experience (although it is probably best to avoid having such a mock examiner for your last practice before the exams).

In all mock exams, try to **seek specific and constructive feedback**. A feedback sheet such as that included at the end of the chapter can help form the basis for this. Do not accept *all* feedback at face value – are the comments accurate, helpful and balanced? If not, seek a further opinion. Ultimately you are seeking to develop a clinical interview and presentation style with which *you* are happy.

It can be quite difficult to make yourself practise in this way. Some find that presenting to a group of other colleagues who are also sitting the exam can be helpful. You will gain from seeing how others present their cases, and they will also learn from you. Try presenting the cases to each other using the formal approach of presenting to *two* 'examiners' as occurs in the exam. Presenting patients who are under the care of a colleague, to someone not directly involved with the case also offers useful experience in an unfamiliar setting. This has the added bonus that it prevents them from asking you unfairly about information that they have prior knowledge of.

Ask friends working in other hospitals to introduce to you their interesting or challenging patients. Always respect the patients right to withhold **consent** for such clinical 'practice', although most patients are perfectly willing to help if asked in a proper manner.

NB   Do not attempt to contact or visit the clinical staff or wards of the hospital you will be examined at. This can lead to disqualification from the exam.

Make sure that you do mock clinical exams on each of the main areas of clinical practice. These are common in practice, and therefore are common in exams:

- Orthopaedics
- Hernias
- Varicose veins
- Neck 'lumps'
- Chronic leg ischaemia
- Hand lesions
- Nerve lesions.

Even mock exams are stressful, but you are far better off learning from your mistakes *before* rather than in the heat of the exam. Knowing that you have an effective presentation style can help you lower your anxiety in the exam setting.

Courses

A lot of short cases are outpatients who are brought to the hospital specifically for the examination. If you cannot get to see a wide range of 'classic' cases in your clinical job, then a clinical course may be helpful.

Exam technique

Some general advice

- Go in and act confidently.
- Passing the clinical is a presentation of *yourself* too.
- Shake the examiners' hands if they initiate this.
- Smile and try to remember the examiners' names.
- Look smart and professional and act competently.
- Be polite but do not come over as too eager to please.
- Make eye contact with *both* examiners as you start presenting, and subsequently.
- Avoid looking at the floor if you don't know something. If the examiners enquire about something that you have forgotten to ask about, say that you would 'normally have enquired about this but have forgotten to', and why it would be important *in this case*.

- Try to appear human by showing (positive) aspects of your personality.
- Be clear and confident.
- Be interesting.

Your approach to the patient

- **Be formal and polite**. Always introduce yourself properly to each patient before proceeding. Ask if you may perform the examination asked of you by the examiners.
- **Talk to the patient in the way that you normally would**. Would you normally address them as 'Sir' or 'Madam' six times while examining the groin? Avoid overfamiliarity. Don't use first names – this will annoy some examiners.
- **Show concern for the patient's comfort**.
- **Enquire if the patient has any pain before proceeding**. This may target your approach and shows that you wish to avoid unnecessary discomfort to the patient.
- **Position the patient correctly** for the particular examination you wish to carry out (e.g. stand *behind* the patient to examine cervical lymph nodes).
- **Be careful with your terminology** in front of the patient when referring to cancer or other emotive subjects such as HIV. You should communicate that you have a proper concern for the patient's welfare.
- After the examination of each patient is complete, ensure that the patient is comfortable and offer to help replace any items of clothing you have removed for the examination.
- The key is to **be calm, respectful, considerate and professional**.

What to do when asked to examine a patient

All necessary equipment will be provided at the correct time and in the correct place. Bear in mind that certain items of equipment will have been put there for a reason (e.g. a stethoscope left by the bedside of a patient with an abdominal mass). Essential equipment *you* should bring includes a pen that works (plus a spare) and a watch with a second hand.

When asked to perform an examination, **listen very carefully to the question**. Many candidates do not, and achieve only a combination of precious time wasted and an irritated examiner. Do not answer the question you would *like* to have been asked instead of the question that *was* asked.

Start by examining the system indicated by the examiner's question unless the examiner has stated specifically that you do otherwise. Remember: **a good doctor is a good observer**. When asked to examine a patient's legs, for instance, noticing that the shoes by the bed have a shoe raise will lead you to think of how to demonstrate the difference between true and apparent leg length inequality and their causes.

Example 1

'Please examine this patient's gastrointestinal system.'

Do a full abdominal examination, starting with the patient's hands, also looking for eye signs, perioral signs etc.

Example 2

'Show me how you would examine for ascites.'

Here, the abdomen should be examined initially for ascites – gentle palpation to exclude areas of tenderness and percussion for detecting shifting dullness and fluid thrill. Do this, but do not hesitate to go on to look for other signs you may think relevant, unless you are interrupted. The intelligent candidate would also have spotted the liver palms and spider naevi on the chest and would volunteer to examine the patient further (e.g. for hepatosplenomegaly). **Be alert to additional signs.**

You will not be failed for being thorough in your examination but **if prompted to move on to a specific area, do so quickly**. You have made your point about being thorough and they are trying to save time by guiding you to where the signs are to be found. Moving on allows you to score more points: the examiners are *not* trying to catch you out.

If you have been asked to examine one system it is quite in order, having done what you have been asked, to **extend your examination to look for other relevant physical signs**. This shows that you understand the significance of your findings and are able to think on your feet, and conveys the impression that you are a knowledgeable and thinking clinician. If you have examined a patient with arthritic hands, looking at the elbows for rheumatoid nodules or patches of psoriasis may help you to diagnose the problem more accurately. In a patient with upper lobe signs on chest examination, a quick look for Horner's syndrome or wasting of the small muscles of the hand shows that you are alert to the possibility of a Pancoast tumour. Always ask yourself if there is anything else you would normally look for in this situation?

Remember that certain organs or conditions demand specific examination techniques, for example:

- Hernias – stand the patient up
- The thyroid – ask the patient to swallow
- The submandibular gland – do a bimanual examination
- Lumps – transilluminate
- Hepatomegaly – look for clubbing, jaundice, spider naevi etc.

Summary

- Perform a thorough **examination of the primary system related to the presenting complaint**.
- A swift professional **general examination should cover all systems** but look particularly for signs of **complications** of the primary disorder and for **evidence corroborating** your diagnosis.
- Take note of (and later mention) obvious clues (e.g. a leg prosthesis): it is surprisingly common to omit these things.

- Use specific examination procedures as required. If appropriate, suggest that you would go on to perform an internal examination as part of your usual practice but *do not* undertake this in the exam.

The spot diagnosis

Occasionally the examiner will require you to do a limited examination or indeed no more examination other than inspection, especially if time is running out. You may be asked:

- For a diagnosis
- To provide an explanation of the apparent abnormality
- To describe associated symptoms or signs
- To provide a differential diagnosis for the abnormality you can see
- To suggest further tests or treatment.

Answering the questions

Tell the examiner what you have heard, seen and felt. You should explain your findings and what you think they mean, and if possible arrive at a diagnosis. **Start with the simple and more common suggestions and not the rarities**.

You should also mention relevant physical signs that you did *not* find which you might have *expected* to find. For example, in a patient with a central abdominal mass it would be pertinent to mention that there was no pulsation and no bruit, or in the case of a scrotal swelling that there was no cough impulse or no transillumination. This shows that you are aware of the differential diagnosis.

Even if you think that you are doing badly, carry on. If a particular case has not gone well try to put it behind you and approach each case as if it is the first.

Interpreting investigations

It is not uncommon either in the short cases or in the viva to be presented with the results of further investigations. These may include the following:

- Radiographs/radioisotope scans/magnetic resonance imaging /computerized tomograms
- Urine, haematology and biochemistry results
- Blood gas results
- Microbiology results.

The interpretation of these requires the factual knowledge that you will have already learnt for the MCQs. Being presented with a radiological examination, however, can make even good candidates unsettled. As in the clinical examination, you need to learn a systematic approach to the description and identification of radiological abnormalities.

Don't know what the abnormality *is*?
You may be able to see an abnormality, but not know what it is. Don't give up – lateral thinking is required:

- Listen to the question carefully: **are there any hints in the question?**
- Sometimes **you may be able to anticipate what the investigation shows** from the facts you already know or from information you are given. This is especially important if the investigation is that of the patient you have just examined. (For example, if, having examined a patient with an old midline scar, colostomy and hepatomegaly, you are given the abdominal CT scan the hepatic lesions would be much more likely to be metastatic than abscesses.)
- Remember that it may be something that you have never seen, but have heard described, **go with your hunches**: if you think, 'so *that's* what it looks like!' you are probably right.

Can't see an abnormality at *all*?
You may not be able to see an abnormality at all when you first see the investigation. Don't give up:

- **Beware of problems not associated with an obvious prime pathology** (e.g. gas under the diaphragm, fractures, transposed or reversed X-rays, a different patient name from the one given on the investigation).

- Carefully and **systematically go through your standard approach** to the interpretation of X-rays, CT scans, MRIs etc. The abnormality will often become obvious but you will gain marks by talking through your approach even if you miss an abnormality.

The diagnosis

If you have made the diagnosis, consider the following while you complete your examination:

- The relevant positive and negative findings
- Your differential diagnosis and the reasons for this
- Your planned investigations
- Your planned management
- An estimate of prognosis
- What you would tell the patient or their relatives (with the patient's consent)
- Possible complications of the diagnosed condition and pro-posed treatment.

When presenting the differential diagnosis, remember that there may be no single right answer. 'You could start with a phrase such as: 'There are a number of possibilities which include . . . '. If it is obvious, however, state what you think the diagnosis is. The examiners' summary of the case includes only key relevant details. Do not automatically assume that they have some vital piece of information that you have not discovered. It is import-ant to remember that you may know as many details as the examiners.

If, in your revision you have pre-prepared a list of 'standardized' differential diagnoses for the common presenting complaints that you come across, these can help you to remember the range of diagnostic possibilities. Having these to fall back on can be a great help if anxiety levels are high and you are finding it difficult to think effectively during the exam. Do remember, however, only to bring these up if you *really are* considering them for this particular case.

It is also important to be adaptable and flexible. Carefully consider any suggestions the examiners make to *you* about diagnosis, etc. Do not reject this out of hand, but show that you can consider the relevant evidence for and against a particular diagnostic possibility. If what they say throws you, remember (and tell the examiners) that all you can comment on is the evidence that you found during your examination. **Never guess** – it is better to admit that you cannot feel the spleen (while showing that you know how to position the patient properly to maximize your chances of feeling it) than to guess. The examiners are not interested in guesses, even if they happen to be right, but are looking for a professional and competent approach.

Your investigations

Think out in advance which other investigations might be appropriate. These could include:

- **Laboratory tests** that are likely to be easily available. State which and why. **Know what these are done for** and the relevance of any abnormality (e.g. a full blood count to exclude the possibility of anaemia etc.)
- **Simple radiological tests** (e.g. a chest X-ray)
- **Confirmatory tests** (ultrasound, bronchoscopy, computerized tomography etc.).

You may be asked early on for a specific **definitive test**, or what investigation you would choose if you could choose only one. For example, in a patient with an acutely ischaemic foot you would want an angiogram as your *principal* investigation (although you would also perform baseline blood investigations, ECG, chest X-ray etc.). Use your common sense. Say what you would do *in practice*.

Presenting to the examiners

- Smile. Try to make appropriate eye contact at an early point.

- Be careful to listen to the question you have been asked and do not leap into a recital of the full history and examination.
- Although one examiner will be asking questions at any one time, you should answer to both examiners as it is the *other* examiner who is marking you on that question.
- Do not be worried if a third examiner is sitting in the background. He or she is a trainee examiner. They will make no contribution at all to your final mark, which is decided by the other two examiners alone.
- Be polite to the examiners, but do not come over as too eager to please. Too much obsequience or the use of 'sir' is unwise.
- If asked for a summary, present the case as though you were the specialist registrar on the consultant's ward round.
- Be prepared to be interrupted. Examiners are asked *not* to let the candidate recite a full history, but instead to encourage them to pursue problem-orientated questions.
- Can you see the wood for the trees? Present the key findings and salient features of the case.

Exam difficulties

The overriding thing to have in mind is that the patients chosen for the exams will be appropriate for the level of exam you are sitting. Sometimes patients may seem very complex. You can still pass the exam by keeping calm and concentrating on technique.

The Royal Colleges advise participating hospitals against using so-called classic 'museum cases' in the MRCS examination and prefer to use cases which test the candidate's clinical skills rather than their recall for the outstandingly obscure. If you *do* come across a rarity, then keep calm and work from common sense and first principles. You cannot be expected to have seen *everything* before but must be able to remain logical. Using effective and well-practised examination techniques can help you to come through this safely.

Remember, if you feel you have made mistakes:

- You are **marked over the full exam** and can make up lost ground. **It is the impression that you make over *all* the cases that counts** and a good performance in one case can make up for a poor showing in another.
- **It is a popular misconception that you have to get all the diagnoses correct and that a single error will fail you the exam**.
- Examiners are primarily looking for competence in clinical examination and a considerate and thoughtful approach. If the examiners start asking you difficult questions or pushing you, take heart – you are doing well and they are trying to find out how good you are rather than whether you should just pass the exam.
- Never leave the exam or give up part of the way through the examination day. Too many candidates who have done this would have passed. Challenge any catastrophic predictions and keep going. **Keep your nerve**. At the very least you will gain useful 'live' examination practice which will stand you in good stead for any future applications. At best you will pass.

Key points

✔ **Keep calm** and always take each short case on its own merits. You may think you have done badly but you really don't know, so don't give up – **keep going**.

✔ **Listen very carefully to the question**.

✔ **State the diagnosis** or a differential diagnosis.

✔ When giving a differential diagnosis try to **list the most likely diagnosis for that patient first**.

✔ **Give reasons for and against your diagnosis** with your relevant positive and negative findings on examination.

✔ Plan your **investigations and management** according to your differential diagnosis.

✔ **If uncertain as to the diagnosis then present your findings clearly, concisely and honestly** and suggest a

---

(continued)

(continued from previous page)

> differential diagnosis and/or investigations that may
> help to pinpoint the diagnosis.
> ✔ **Be careful with your terminology** in front of the patient
> when referring to cancer or other such emotive
> subjects.
> ✔ Make sure that you come over as **safe, sensible and
> professional**.
> ✔ Try to **answer as if this was an everyday clinical
> situation**.

MOCK CLINICAL EXAM ASSESSMENT SHEET

(Please photocopy and use if you wish.)

Examiner: **Candidate:**

Initial case presentations: The ability to pick out the salient features of the case and present these clearly and coherently should be assessed. The organization of information is particularly important. The assessment of relevant physical factors should be recognised in the mark.

Discussion: Is the differential diagnosis, aetiology, management and prognosis of the case discussed knowledgeably, paying regard to social and psychological factors as well as purely physical approaches?

Professionalism: Polite and professional attitude? The ability to cover the appropriate clinical areas quickly, clearly and efficiently should be assessed.

Overall mark: A general discussion with the candidate would probably be more helpful rather than an overall statement of Pass or Fail.

Comments: Helpful ways to improve presentation and organization of material?

7

The viva

Introduction

The viva attempts to make sure that you have a sound knowledge of the basic surgical sciences, the principles of the practice of surgery and critical care, and that you are clinically safe. It offers the examiners a chance to find out how much you know and, more importantly, to assess whether you can tackle a problem in a calm and logical manner even when the answer is not immediately apparent to you.

You will be expected to answer with a level of knowledge that is reasonable for someone of potential specialist registrar level. Do not be put off if the question is put to you by an examiner who you fear may be a specialist in that area. All that will be expected is for you to have a *reasonable* overall level of knowledge and to understand the general principles involved. The second examiner is marking your answer, and if they feel the question is unreasonable, they will discount it.

Learning for the viva is difficult as it can cover almost any aspect of surgery, but remembering a few general principles will help you with this part of the exam:

- **You are not expected to know everything**. Do not try to bluff your way through this part of the exam; instead, try to come over as honest and thoughtful. Practice is essential to make sure that you are able to communicate what you would do in a variety of clinical situations in a clear and structured way.
- There will be two examiners interviewing you: both will give you marks. It is important that you should address your remarks to both examiners and not just the one asking the

question. There may be a third person present, who will be a trainee MRCS examiner. They will not be involved in the interview itself and will not contribute to your final mark.

Content of the viva

Basic sciences

There is always a strong emphasis on anatomy, physiology and pathology. These may be asked either in isolation or related to a clinical topic:

- Know the anatomy involved in common surgical procedures (e.g. hernia repair, hip replacement etc.[1])
- Know the physiology of critical care of the surgical patient (e.g. shock, fluid balance etc.)
- Know the pathological appearances of common surgical problems (e.g. inflammatory bowel disease, lymphoma etc.)

You must have in-depth knowledge of these subjects with particular reference to the surgical topics below.

Important surgical topics

- **Acute surgical problems**, both diagnostic and therapeutic. Know your **surgical emergencies**[2]. This should not be a problem as it is closely linked to your job. You have been doing this for years on the wards and in A & E. Say what you would do in practice.
- **Outpatient clinic scenarios**: intended to show if you are happy with the collation of all available clues and medical knowledge in an effective manner.
- **Investigation material**: blood results, for example, may be the focus of a question.
- **Current themes in the literature**: a number of MRCS examiners believe that the importance of this component is overemphasized by many candidates. Be aware of current trends, however, and be prepared to discuss them with a reasonable level of knowledge.

You should read through recent Editorial leaders in the *British Journal of Surgery* and the *Lancet* as well as at least a year's issues of *Surgery*. This can help highlight current issues in clinical practice and 'hot' topics. You do not need to read every article in great detail but it will help you to be aware of what is topical. It may also be helpful to read the medical sections in the Sunday papers as these often deal with new advances and controversies and are a quick way of keeping abreast of what is going on.

Be prepared to answer an open question (e.g., *'What do you think is the most important clinical development in the last ten years?'* or *'What paper that you have read recently has changed your clinical practice?'*). Prepare for this type of question. It is worth the trouble and can change a nightmare question into a joy. A warning, though – do not argue. You can give your answer and your reasons for that answer, but do not antagonize your examiners. You may win the battle but risk losing the war.

Management plans
You may be asked about some of the following areas:

- If asked what your **immediate management on admission of a patient** would be, start with the steps necessary to ensure the **patient's immediate safety** as if you were the receiving surgeon (**A**irway, **B**reathing, **C**irculation, if appropriate)
- Say simple things first. For example, you would offer **supportive measures** for a patient with appendicitis – analgesia, antiemetics, nil-by-mouth, i.v. fluids etc.
- Simple measures include **relevant communications with the nursing staff or other ward professionals** to investigate the patient's mobility, make observations, regulate fluid intake, or diet etc.
- **Investigations** (e.g. angiogram or contrast enema)
- **Medical intervention with drugs** (e.g. the use of mannitol in head injuries, radioiodine in the treatment of thyrotoxicosis)
- **Surgical intervention** (e.g. embolectomy, laparotomy)
- **Rehabilitation** (physical, social, and financial)

- Indications for seeking the **opinion of a doctor in another specialty**
- Assessment by a physiotherapist or an occupational therapist may also sometimes be helpful in assessment and treatment of the patient
- **Provision of information** – education, instructions and advice for the patient and their relatives may be important
- **Psychological and social considerations** – the illness may have not only biological implications, but may result in a change in home, occupation or financial security. How is the person likely to cope with their illness? What are their concerns and fears about the future?
- **Planned discharge from hospital** if an inpatient. Will the patient/relatives be able to manage at home or will they need **support**? This may include referral for district nurse, hospice, social services or Macmillan nurses etc.
- **Support for the patient and their family** is always important, particularly in chronic or life-threatening conditions. Indicate what you might tell the patient or family (with the patient's consent) if they ask about the possible outcome of this illness.

Prognosis

Offer your experience, not just the theory. Consider both the *classic prognosis* of this condition as summarized in books and research papers and the *specific features* of the patient which affect prognosis in *this* case. Try to give the main indicators for a good or bad prognosis in the patient you have seen. This might include:

- Previous history
- The type and extent of surgery carried out
- Patient compliance (e.g. with physiotherapy after anterior cruciate ligament reconstruction, or with bandaging, medication etc.).

Emphasize that the decision on your treatment plan (symptomatic, supportive or curative) will depend on the prognosis.

Preparation for the viva

Common questions

Certain topics lend themselves very well to viva questions and certain questions come up time and time again. You should try to spot such areas and commit them to memory, so that they can be reproduced easily and reliably on the day of the exam. It cannot be stressed enough how much can be asked about the basic sciences. These questions can come up in a variety of guises.

Examples of basic science questions

- *Describe the anatomical landmarks for a thyroidectomy* – anatomy
- *What are the principles involved in preoperative 'workup' of the thyrotoxic patient?* – physiology
- *What are the causes of a thyroid mass?* – pathology

There is a lot of factual knowledge to be absorbed. Try using Mind Maps® to produce answers for the common questions. If revising in a group, swap revision notes to build up a library of quick reference material to use in the weeks leading up to the viva. The night before the viva is not the time to be reaching for the *Oxford Textbook of Surgery* for the first time.

Here is a list of suggestions on how to identify the important areas:

- The areas examined are included in the information booklets on the MRCS syllabus produced by the Colleges. It is useful to look at *all* the Colleges' booklets to get the full range of topics
- You will be able to predict questions from textbooks[3], distance-learning course manuals etc.
- Discuss the exam with colleagues who have passed the MRCS – they may be able to remember old exam questions

• Courses specifically tailored to the exam provide useful 'crammer' revision sessions and act as pointers to the types of questions you may be asked.

Mock vivas

It is important to practise mock vivas. A useful source of questions for practice are viva revision books. Many candidates find answering viva questions surprisingly difficult, simply because they have not become familiar with the technique. Basically, tell the examiner what *you* would do in such a case in your own clinical practice. After all, you have been solving similar problems whilst 'on call' and on the wards for the last few years. Be sensible and safe, and you will pass. Candidates' nerves are usually at their worst waiting for the exam and you may find that you feel a lot better once the exam is under way. Using the techniques outlined in the next sections and making sure that you have practised this style of examination before the actual day should boost your confidence and settle your nerves.

Viva techniques

Many candidates faced with a question about a topic with which they are unfamiliar become anxious and lose the structure to their answer. They often know all that is required and yet feel that they should know something more. **Structure your answer** so that limited information can be presented in a meaningful manner. Regular practice in answering questions will significantly improve your ability to structure and present answers. Learn to **communicate what you know clearly and concisely**.

The examiners have questions prepared for the viva. They depend on the candidate, however, for the follow-up questions. If you list a rare cause of a symptom, be prepared to be asked about it. In trying to convey all the information that you know it is easy not to think this far ahead. This can be improved with practice. Answering in the viva is a little like answering questions in court: think where every response may lead and try to **direct the questions towards your stronger areas**.

A number of techniques are central to answering viva questions effectively:

- It is essential to be **systematic and organized** in your approach
- Do not restrict your answers so that you only answer one part of the question. It is easy to make the mistake of answering on only one aspect of the problem, so heading down a 'blind alley' and running out of things to say. **Keep your thinking broad and at a basic level initially**
- **Do not say too much** – you may talk yourself into trouble! Never open a door that you are not prepared to walk through
- Try to **keep your answers simple to start with** and then build on this foundation with additional knowledge
- Try to avoid lengthy pauses.

You need to have a clear opening, a structured main section, and a clear ending to your answer.

The opening
Try to avoid a lengthy pause. Your answer should have a clear opening. The following three approaches may help you to get started and to structure your answer.

1. Point out the main thrust of the question
You can gain thinking time by saying what the main thrust of the question involves (thinking out loud).

What are the main issues raised by the question?

- Diagnosis, investigation or management?
- Conservative, medical or surgical management?
- Patient issues (compliance etc.)?

2. Suggest what further information might be required
Do you need any more information? (And if so, where from?)

- To make the diagnosis?
- To decide on treatment? What are the benefits and risks of treatment?
- To assess the impact on the patient?

These two approaches show the examiners that you can **pick out the key points quickly** and that you have a firm grasp of the essentials of care.

3. Talk yourself into the situation

Another way of helping you gain valuable thinking time is to talk yourself into the situation, showing the examiners that you grasp the key features of the case. For example, you might begin, 'If I was asked to go and see this case in A&E, I would check that the patient had been fully resuscitated and that baseline investigations had been ordered . . . ' Some people find this approach to be most effective when they use visual imagery as they talk about how they would deal with the situation. **This approach is often particularly helpful if you are feeling quite anxious**.

Do not begin to answer each question in exactly the same way. This may annoy and frustrate the examiners.

The main part of your answer

Perhaps the best way to understand what is required in this part of your answer would be to summarize the features of good and bad practice.

Qualities of a 'bad' answer:

- The answer lacks structure and is presented badly with comments such as 'I meant to say . . . oh yes, and also' etc.
- Eye contact with the examiner is avoided by staring at the floor when the answer is not known.
- The candidate clearly lacks confidence and comes over as someone who cannot make a decision or show effective clinical judgement. They have no answer to follow-up questions which seem to floor them.
- A list of responses is given which takes no account of the relative frequency and importance of the condition's investigations/treatments.

- A major cause/feature is completely left out.
- There is no definite end point to the answer, which rambles on ineffectively.

Try to avoid suggesting increasingly rare causes towards the end of the answer as this invites follow-up questions about the things you know least. *Never* say something like 'There are ten causes of an enlarged spleen' – it will not come over well if you can only remember six! Never be tempted to lie in the exam and say that you have done something you have not, or read an article you have never seen. You may find the article in question was written by one of the examiners!

Qualities of a 'good' answer:

- There is an effective structure to the answer
- Eye contact with the examiners is made, in a non-challenging way
- The candidate speaks clearly and confidently, showing a professional manner
- The list of responses covers all the important and common conditions
- There is a clear end-point to the answer
- Try to demonstrate confidence and an organized mind – you will gain thinking time by using a structured approach. A clear structure also means that the examiners will not insist on an exhaustive list and excuses you from having to rank your answers in order of frequency or importance. You can always add comments such as 'I think that malignancy is the most *likely* cause in this case because . . . ' to clarify this. Interesting information such as less common causes can be held back to satisfy follow-up questions. The answer should come to a clear end, when you should look up, waiting for the next question or instruction.

Here are two examples of typical questions and suggestions. Structure your response.

Example 1

'What are the causes of an enlarged spleen?'

It is impossible to answer this question well without structuring your response. The candidate who begins to reel off an infinitely long list of possible causes, starting with the most obscure, will exasperate examiners. Always think of the question as if it ended with, *'Please list these with the most commonly encountered first'*. You could begin your answer with a statement such as 'Several disease processes can cause an enlarged spleen, for example': and then go on to list the most common:

- **Infective** causes, such as malaria, glandular fever etc.
- **Malignancies**, such as . . .
- **Haematological causes**, such as . . .
- **Portal hypertension**, secondary to . . .
- **Storage disorders**, such as . . .
- **Cardiovascular problems**, such as . . . .

Example 2

'What do you know about neurofibromatosis?'

You might structure your answer like this:

- Neurofibromatosis is an uncommon, autosomal dominant, inherited condition.
- It exists in two major forms, Type 1 and Type 2.
- Patients often present with dermatological features, such as . . .
- Complications include . . . .

Reducing anxiety

When candidates are nervous they tend to talk too fast. This reduces thinking time substantially and suggests a lack of confidence. Anxiety also makes structuring answers difficult and you may overwhelm the examiner with information. This can lead to mistakes and confusion and will probably irritate your examiners. When asked a question, **take a few seconds to think about the answer**. Try to talk slowly and pause between each sentence of your answer.

Answer with confidence. If a candidate appears underconfident or unsure, the examiner will feel that they do not know their subject well. Certainty comes with practice and knowledge. **You can still be confident even if you don't know the answer to a question**: say *where* you would go for the information or *who* you would discuss the case with, for further clarification. For example, if you do not know what drugs you can safely prescribe in pregnancy it would be quite reasonable to say, 'I would contact Pharmacy and Drug Information and ask for further information'. Sometimes, in practice, it would be appropriate to discuss a clinical problem with your boss or seek a specialist opinion – if so, say so. The MRCS candidate is not expected to know *everything*. If you do not know the answer, admit that you do not (though try not to do this too often).

Confidence is very important but **overconfidence is potentially disastrous**. If you are overconfident and try to bluff your way through a subject you know little about, you are potentially dangerous in the clinical situation. **You are more likely to worry the examiners if you give the impression that you believe you can treat *everything, all of the time***.

If you find that the questions are getting more difficult, do not be disheartened. The examiners interview a lot of candidates and will *enjoy* a candidate who is doing well. They may ask increasingly difficult questions in order to determine just how good the candidate is. In this part of the exam, if the examiners seem to be building up the pressure it is because the examinee is doing well, not because they are doing badly. **Do not get the wrong impression**. Candidates often worry quite unnecessarily.

The examiner may well ask a question which they do not really expect the candidate to be able to answer. The purpose of this is to determine *how* the candidate thinks and how they approach the unknown. The exam is not designed to test only the recall of factual information, but to ensure that the candidate knows how to approach a patient, knows how to think through a problem and how to deal with the unexpected – in essence, how to be a good clinician.

If the examiners appear to disagree with you, be prepared to consider other possibilities. Feel able to discuss other diagnostic or treatment options, but never get into an argument. If you think that you *are* correct, you should review the reasons for and against each of the possibilities and the reasons why you wish, for the time being, to stick to your first decision. Always show that if more information were to become available, or the condition of the patient changed, you would be willing to reconsider. **Never let yourself become angry or confrontational with an examiner**. If you do this, you *will* fail.

Broad thinking

Another reason why some candidates seem to grind to a premature halt is the use of narrow thinking. Any question is likely to elicit a few instant and obvious answers from a candidate. Full marks will not be gained, however, unless other possibilities or important aspects of the case are also mentioned. For example, the candidate may know about the whole range of consequences of a condition, but only mention one or two. You must take the view that 'if they're asking for six points then I know six points'. To access the rest of the information the examiner is looking for, you must **make a conscious effort to broaden your thinking**. These two suggestions may help you to achieve this:

1. Consider what area of your knowledge you are using to answer the question. You may be able to add to your answer by **switching to other areas of knowledge**. Consciously broadening your approach to include other subspecialty areas can help. For example, you may be approaching the question from the point of view of orthopaedics – a switch to thinking from the point of view of rehabilitation might stimulate further ideas (and further marks).

2. **Think of the headings of a 'surgical sieve'.** This is particularly useful in questions about aetiology. There are many sieves – use the one that you can remember. (See Chapter 8 for more information on the use of sieves.)

These techniques aim to encourage you to think more broadly and help you to **access information that you already know**.

The principles of effective answering of viva questions are illustrated in this example:

Example

How would you manage a 50-year-old man with a history of rectal bleeding?

You should be able to provide a full and extensive answer, but as soon as it is apparent that you are knowledgeable in this area, the examiners are likely to guide you with leading questions which can produce an answer more like a 'tennis match' than a monologue. The following illustrates one possible answer to this question. It is unlikely that you will be able to offer the *full* answer: the examiners are likely to interrupt and guide you into specific areas. This is normal, but can be disconcerting. You should try to lead the questioning into areas in which you are knowledgeable and feel comfortable.

Possible answer

- First you must examine the question and define what it means, both for the examiners and yourself.
- Describe how your immediate action would depend on the amount of blood lost PR and on the clinical condition of the patient (e.g. if he was hypotensive and tachycardic, the first priority would be correction of his circulatory collapse with IV access and fluids).

(continued)

(continued from previous page)

- Say that you would make a thorough examination starting with 'ABC', including pulse, blood pressure, appearance and examination of the abdomen (including PR examination).
- Start your assessment with a full history, including family history for GI malignancy, use of non-steroidal drugs or warfarin, alteration in bowel habit, pain, etc.
- Demonstrate that you would be aware of factors that may mask the severity of the patient's condition (e.g. a patient on beta-blockers with a normal pulse rate or a patient on steroids with a hidden perforation).
- Comment on the investigations you would order, pointing out that the first haemoglobin reading may be normal, despite a significant bleed, as haemodilution has not yet occurred.
- Say that you would order repeated observations to monitor any changes in the patient's condition.
- Discuss how further investigations and their urgency would depend on the clinical progression of the patient. Proctoscopy and rigid sigmoidoscopy can be carried out as bedside procedures. Urgent endoscopy or even laparotomy may be necessary if the patient deteriorates rapidly.
- The examiners will expect you to be able to draw up a list of differential diagnoses. Use a surgical sieve to remind you to include neoplasia (GI malignancy), inflammatory bowel disease, vascular abnormalities (e.g. haemorrhoids, angiodysplasia, AV malformation), etc.
- Finally, but importantly, show that you are aware of the impact of illness on the patient and his family and friends. PR bleeding is very stressful for patients who may be scared by what is happening and the possibility of surgery. Show briefly that you are aware of this and would address such concerns in your management plan.

In summary, the examiners are attempting to determine your level of knowledge and your ability to process information in a way that is appropriate to the *normal* practice of surgery. The best approach, therefore, is to try to forget that it is an exam and imagine that you are being given this information in an everyday clinical situation.

Key points

✔ Presentation should be calm and structured.
✔ Be aware of the range of possible questions.
✔ Practice will help.
✔ Be seen to be clinically sensible and safe in the clinical setting.
✔ Answer the question asked, not the one you would want to be asked.
✔ Say what you would do in practice.
✔ Use broad thinking.
✔ Organize your answer clearly.
✔ Gain thinking time by considering what further information you require and what the key issues are. 'Talking yourself into' the clinical scenario may also help.
✔ Do not be argumentative.
✔ Where appropriate, say that you would seek information or advice from others with more experience in the area.

REFERENCES

1). Kirk RM (2000) *General Surgical Operations*, 4th edn. Churchill Livingstone: Edinburgh.

2). Monson J, Duthie G, O'Malley K (1999) *Surgical Emergencies*. Blackwell Science: Oxford.

3). Mokbel KM (1996) *Operative Surgery and Surgical Topics for the FRCS/MRCS*, Revised edn. Libra Pharm. Ltd. – Petroc Press.

Just before the exams

This chapter summarizes many of the principles already discussed in the book and will give you some additional useful techniques to help you to structure your answers. If you have just 15 minutes before the exam, this chapter may be the one to read.

There are many people who are well respected in their hospitals and who are excellent and knowledgeable clinicians who, much to the surprise of their colleagues, fail the clinical exam. Many of them will have underachieved because of poor *performance*. They have not been able to communicate what they know to the examiners in an organized and structured way.

Many examiners think that being able to perform effectively in stressful situations (such as a difficult viva) prepares a candidate for dealing with stressful clinical situations (e.g. major trauma). Whether or not this is true, it remains the case that a candidate who is able to present calmly and professionally is more likely to stand out as someone who should pass.

It can be very disheartening to go into the clinical or viva brimming over with factual information and to end up being unable to communicate what you know. One of the greatest problems for candidates is remaining calm under pressure. Anxiety can make you flustered and present information that is disorganized, unstructured, or frankly incorrect. While some people are natural performers others may perform badly, either by appearing to have nothing to say or by giving answers that they would not dream of considering during their normal work.

It is important that you give careful thought to how *you* perform under pressure. There are several ways to practise calm and structured presentation. These encourage you to familiarize yourself with presenting under pressure, so that the exam is not the first time you have to 'perform' when anxious. One of the most effective ways of reducing exam anxiety is to have learned how to structure your presentation.

Structuring your answer

You must have an effective opening, a well-thought-out middle section, and a clear end to your presentation.

Effective openings

Try to avoid long pauses which might give the appearance that you are struggling to answer. Consider using one of these three opening gambits to help you to structure your response and gain some thinking time.

1. Mention the 'key issues': quickly summarize the important elements of the answer. For example, 'This question raises a number of key issues such as:

- Screening / epidemiology
- Clinical assessment
- Immediate clinical management (including surgical approaches)
- Issues of consent

or

- Issues of postoperative or ongoing care.

2. State what further information you would need to clarify the diagnosis or to decide on management. This might include the results of further X-rays, blood tests etc. Always state what *you* would do and *why* you would do it. (Avoid just providing long rambling lists of tests that are not relevant in this particular case, however.)

3. 'Talk yourself into the situation' – this is particularly effective if you are asked to comment on a practical clinical problem. For example, you could begin: 'If I was asked to review this patient on the ward, after a brief initial assessment, I would read the clinical notes, speak to the ward staff, and then . . . .'

Try to vary your opening so that you do not use the same form of words for every answer as this could irritate the examiners.

The middle section

After producing a clear opening, maintain the structure of your answer with a well-planned middle section.

Organise your thoughts. The examiners often ask questions that have several possible answers, e.g. 'So what could be the causes of jaundice in this patient?'. To answer this you are required not only to know the causes of jaundice but also to know how to organize this list in a way relevant to the case presented to you. Many people find this hard work, but with practice and by remembering a few simple principles we shall summarize later in the chapter, you should find the organization of this information easier.

Consider your character and presentation style. (Ask a few trusted colleagues.) Try to show the *positive* aspects of your personality: a quiet, introspective candidate can be misinterpreted as lacking factual knowledge or confidence. On the other hand, an overexuberant extrovert could be seen as brash or arrogant. It will require practice to change, but an introvert can work on projecting themselves more forcibly and extroverts can 'tone down'. If you know that you can be quite shy, use techniques such as looking at an object which is at eye-level and between or just behind the examiners. Even if you don't make direct eye contact, this action will help you to avoid being interpreted as someone lacking in confidence who stares at the ground all the time.

Try to appear sensible and competent. You need to keep the main content of your answer broad and avoid going down a blind alley, addressing only one component of the answer. Resist the temptation to suggest answers which you cannot substantiate.

Finishing your answer

Summarize the answer in two or three sentences: this lets the examiner know that you have finished, and not just pausing for thought. Have a clear ending and try not to just grind to halt!

Sieves and other reminders

There are several methods you can use to broaden the scope of your answers. At undergraduate level, learning is based on a pathological classification of disease. The diagnostic approach, based on symptoms and signs, is nearer to working practice. You must first cast your net wide over all possible diagnoses and then progressively eliminate some and confirm others. A number of techniques can be used to help you do this, and several aides-mémoires are listed below. Ask your colleagues for theirs to see if they have any tricks that you can use.

The anatomical sieve

Is the problem due to a problem with a superficial or a deep structure? For example, an abdominal mass may originate from a variety of sources.

1. The abdominal wall, including:
   - Skin
   - Subcutaneous tissue
   - Muscle and connective tissue
   - Peritoneum.

2. The viscera, including:
   - Gastrointestinal tract
   - Solid organs
   - Vascular structures.

Another method would be to group organize your list into organ systems (e.g. cardiovascular, gastrointestinal, genito-urinary etc.).

The surgical sieve

When faced by a lesion, consider its possible aetiology by asking yourself whether its origin might be:

- Inherited
- Congenital
- Metabolic
- Infective
- Inflammatory
- Vascular
- Neoplastic
- Toxic or drug-related
- Degenerative
- Traumatic
- Nutritional
- Other.

Overlay the surgical sieve with the anatomical sieve in order to use this approach most effectively. Try this technique for yourself, using the topic, 'Causes of haemoproteinuria'. Spend a few minutes considering this and writing down your answers. A possible answer is provided at the end of the chapter. This answer is neither exclusive nor intended as an example of perfection. Ultimately, you must present your own answer in your own words. You need to communicate to the examiners that you have considered all the relevant diagnostic factors in your assessment. Remember, however, that when you present your findings or diagnosis you should be able to back them up and give *reasons* for your conclusions. You must not suggest a category from the surgical sieve if you do not have an example to hand.

Another way to structure your answer is to ask yourself these questions for each topic – who?, what?, where?, when?, why? and how?

Questions often begin 'How would you manage . . . ?'. The answer could be structured around these headings:

- History
- Examination
- Investigations
- Differential diagnosis
- Initial treatment
- Special investigations
- Diagnosis
- Definitive treatment
- Prognosis
- Follow-up.

A difficult question that often throws even good candidates starts 'Tell me about . . . '. This gives you the opportunity to show the examiner how much you know about a topic (e.g. 'Tell me about bowel cancer.'). Without structure, however, the information will not flow in a coherent and sensible way. In order to answer this broad sort of question, you will need to organize your answer. One approach might be to consider the following headings, using mnenomics to help you remember them:

Heading	Mnemonic
Incidence	*In*
Age	*A*
Sex	*Surgeon's*
Geography	*Gown*
Aetiology	*A*
Pathology	*Physician*
– Macroscopic	*May*
– Microscopic	*Make*
Symptoms and signs	*Some*
Surgery	*Steady*
Prognosis	*Progress*

Everyone has different memory systems (Mind Maps®, mnemonics etc.) – the important point to stress is that you must test your own systems in exam conditions. It is no good remembering a mnemonic if you cannot remember the diagnoses that go with it!

Possible answer to 'the causes of haemoproteinuria'

Pre-renal:
- Inherited (haemophilia)
- Infective (sub-acute bacterial endocarditis etc.)
- Vascular (hypertension etc.)

Renal:
- Inherited (polycystic kidneys, Alport's syndrome etc.)
- Congenital (reflux nephropathy etc.)
- Metabolic (diabetes mellitus, hyperuricaemia)
- Infective (tuberculosis, urinary tract infections)
- Inflammatory (systemic lupus erythematosus, polyarteritis nodosa etc.)
- Vascular (arteriovenous malformation etc.)
- Neoplastic (renal cell carcinoma, non-metastatic membranous nephropathy)
- Toxic or drug-related (non-steroidal anti-inflammatory drugs, penicillamine etc.)

Post-renal:
- Congenital (spinal bifida with collecting system abnormalities etc.)
- Metabolic (renal stones etc.)
- Infective (urinary tract infection, cystitis, pyelonephritis etc.)
- Inflammatory (retroperitoneal fibrosis etc.)
- Neoplastic (urothelial tumours or invading tumours etc.)
- Toxic or drug-related (cyclophosphamide etc.)

Appendix 1: What if you fail? – trying again

Siân McIver

> *'You may be disappointed if you fail, but you are doomed if you don't try.'*
>
> Beverley Sills   (b. 1929)
> American opera singer and manager

Failing the exam

The results come out a number of weeks after the MCQ papers for Part I. Even if you think the exam went badly and during these few weeks you have convinced your friends and family that you *know* you have failed and are resolved to retaking at the next sitting, you will perhaps not have convinced *yourself* quite completely of this. Up until that last minute before the 'bad news envelope' hits the hall carpet, there will still be a glimmer of hope that you have passed.

Unfortunately, the truth is that even some of those who felt that the exam had gone well will have failed. There will be those who have laboured long and hard, covering even the most obscure parts of huge tomes in great detail, who will have to go through this dispiriting experience. It is at this point that the most negative and unrealistic thoughts may emerge: 'I'll never pass' or 'My partner will leave me if I have to put them through that again'. Such thoughts are both unhelpful and inaccurate but part of the normal adjustment reaction that will take place. At this point, if you have just failed, try to find someone objective to discuss the clinical cases or viva questions with. You will find that you *do* have strengths and it will be necessary to remind yourself of this. Ask senior colleagues if they have any thoughts as to why you failed. Encourage them to be honest.

Letting other people know the results can be one of the most difficult undertakings, as this may well be the first important exam you have failed. It is worth taking some time over telling the people you care about most so that they can appreciate what a blow this has been to you and can offer you support. At work, try to remember that probably about half of the consultants you work with will also have had to resit this exam at some time (and yet you probably would not be able to tell which ones they were). Colleagues may try to ascertain whether you have passed or not by watching you from a distance before deciding whether to ask. Some may be sympathetic and supportive; for the others, give a short but positive reply.

Failing a postgraduate exam is a major life event and you will be more likely to succeed at a resit attempt if you allow yourself to recover emotionally first. Be kind to yourself, get plenty of sleep and spend some time doing your favourite things. At a practical level there may be things that you have postponed due to the exam that may get in the way of future revision if you don't attend to now. You may need to have central heating fitted or to see some long-neglected relatives, for instance. Now is also the time to sort out your finances – resits are expensive. Make sure that you claim for all the expenses you were entitled to from your first attempt, and remember that some Trusts will pay for revision courses for resit candidates. This is also a good time to get your CV up to date – you may end up applying for a job near the time of your resit and you won't welcome the diversion of sorting it out then. Keep a copy on disc so that when you pass the exam you can just fill in the date. Not only will these things ease the burden on your time nearer the resit, they will also help to restore some perspective to your life. The exam, and even your career, is only *one* part of your life, but it *is* possible to become totally immersed in it and lose sight of other, more important things.

Why did I fail?

Whenever plans go awry it is important to try and find out why it happened. You must evaluate the situation because, if you don't know why things went wrong the first time, it is possible that you may make the same mistakes again. You must be honest with yourself when answering the question 'Why did I fail?'. Most people who fail know exactly why they failed – **learn from your experience**. Could it be that you hadn't looked carefully enough at central areas and concentrated on peripheral subjects? Did you skimp on books or courses? Another possibility may be that you didn't book your study leave early enough and not only did you end up without any time off to revise before the exam, but you were working harder than usual, covering for your more organized colleagues who had booked theirs well in advance. Even those who know the facts of the subjects inside out may fail as a result of poor exam technique.

If these weren't the cause of your failure then you may have to consider the possibility that your result was caused by the simple and catastrophic error of just not working hard enough. In other words, you can plan, organize, timetable, and buy books until it becomes an art form but you do need to leave time to study as well.

Moving on

In order to move on from here you will need to motivate yourself and decide that this really is the direction that you want to go in. It may be that you were sitting the exam for the *wrong reasons* or that you were actually sitting the *wrong exam*, and now may be a good time to review this. If you decide to alter your career direction at this time, make sure that you are making the decision for positive reasons, and not using it as an avoidance strategy. Even if you are sure that you are doing the right exam it may not be the best *time* for you to resit, (e.g. if you are just about to have a new addition to the family). Generally speaking, however, it is probably best to pay for the resit while the information from the last attempt is still fresh in your mind.

Once you have decided to attempt the exam again, dedication is required to revise all over again. Beware of focusing all your efforts on the part of the exam that you failed. It would be very upsetting to pass this with flying colours the next time, only to fail on another part. A revision timetable may help. Not only will it ensure that you cover each topic but it will also mean that you can timetable breaks where you can be free from the guilt of not working. Some people find it helpful to meet with other people who are sitting the exam – a study group – sitting with a large pot of coffee and some chocolate biscuits can really help the information to go in! Check out which study courses are available and apply for these and for private study leave as soon as possible. Consider attending a specific course on examination techniques if you think that the problem is an inability to communicate what you know effectively.

In conclusion, if you fail the exam try to:

- Evaluate the reasons why you failed
- Motivate yourself to press on and do the resit
- Dedicate yourself to the hard work of revision
- Appreciate the importance of exam techniques so that you present what you know to its best effect.

'If you have made mistakes . . . there is always another chance for you . . . you may have a fresh start any moment you choose, for this thing we call "failure" is not the falling down but the staying down.'

Mary Pickford (1893–1979)

American actress

Appendix 2: Mind Maps®

Kevin Appleton

What are Mind Maps® and how can they help with the exam?

You will already be aware of your strengths and weaknesses when it comes to learning for exams. You will probably use techniques that you have (successfully) used over the years. Successful techniques allow you to structure, organize and integrate new information with the information that you already know in order to make learning meaningful. This is important because, particularly with the Part II exam, it is a practical impossibility to read through everything again in the few days before the exam. It is important to focus on key facts, so that these may be concentrated on in order to reduce the amount of reading you have to do when the work is revised.

Common and effective techniques to help you reduce the quantity of information you have to learn include writing short summary notes or using highlighter pens to focus in on key facts. Another less common approach is Mind Mapping®. This is not an approach that everyone will find intuitively appealing, but some people find this approach to be a very helpful way of organizing and learning information.

Mind Maps® are colourful, branching pictures or diagrams that can help your memory, thinking and organization of ideas and information. They can make study more efficient by condensing more facts onto a single sheet so that very large amounts of information may be revised very quickly. In Mind Map® 1 (see page 108) the assessment and treatment of head injury is covered, together with the ways head injury can lead to presentation to the medical services. To maximize the effectiveness of Mind Maps® it is necessary to produce your own so that each sub-heading of the mind map will trigger off associated pieces of information in your own memory. If you had Mind Map® 1 in mind during the short cases or viva, you should be able to answer most questions on this topic.

Mind Maps® work by increasing the cross-connections and associations of stored information in memory. They use images or key words to anchor information and to trigger associations. It is possible to hold entire Mind Maps® in visual memory and they are fun to use, making learning more enjoyable and revision less tedious. By using different modes of memory storage (e.g. factual, visual and colour), they increase the number of ways in which information can be remembered. In comparison, linear text uses only one storage modality.

How to create your own Mind Maps®

It is better to draw Mind Maps® across the horizontal axis of the page as the structure spreads out better this way. Start with a central image or icon. Recalling this from visual memory will trigger your recall of the whole map. Next arrange main headings or key words around this from the centre of the page outwards. Sub-headings, lists and further details can then be added to each branch.

One heading or icon (e.g. head injury, as in Mind Map®1) will come to represent, in your own mind, many other additional responses (subdural, penetrating, etc.). These act as anchors for surrounding text and help you to recall this additional information efficiently. Well organized information should result in an aesthetically pleasing map; poorly organized information will look a mess and will be harder to recall. To structure the content clearly on paper means that it must also be structured clearly in your mind, so that drawing out the diagram is itself an effective means of revision. This is illustrated by Mind Map® 2 (see page 109), which summarizes the use and production of Mind Maps®. You will be able to see how the key elements of the linear text you are now reading can be summarized clearly and concisely on one sheet of paper. This is both information-rich, and very quickly read. If this summarizes this chapter effectively for you, could the technique also be useful for your exam revision?

Because Mind Maps® can summarize large amounts of information into a manageable form, this information can be reviewed very quickly just before the exam. They make it possible to revise the contents of an entire book in a short period of time. Two further examples of Mind Maps® (summarizing postoperative pain management [3] and fracture fixation [4]) have been reproduced on pages 110 and 111.

A full account of the use of Mind Maps® can be found in *The Mind Map Book* by Buzan and Buzan[1].

Please note: The terms Mind Map® and Mind Mapping® are registered trade marks of the Buzan Centres Ltd, Suites 2 and 3, 37 Waterloo Road, Bournemouth BH9 1BD.

REFERENCES

1). Buzan T, Buzan B (1993) *The Mind Map Book*. BBC Books, BBC Enterprises: London.

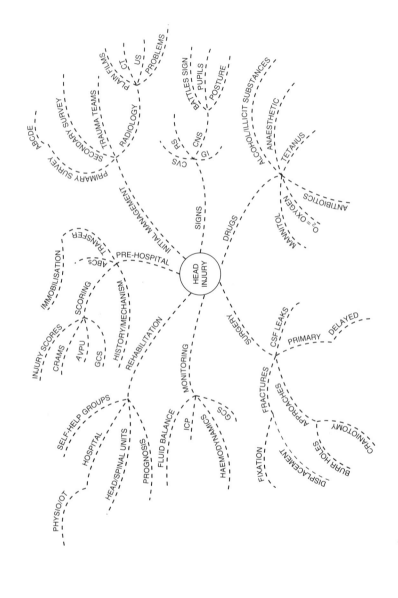

Mind Map®1. Head injury

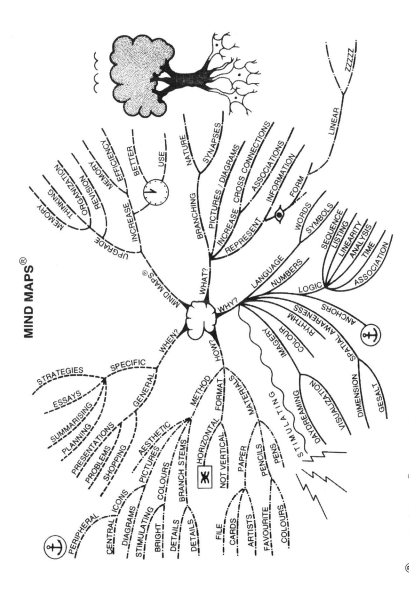

Mind Map®2. Mind Maps® summarized

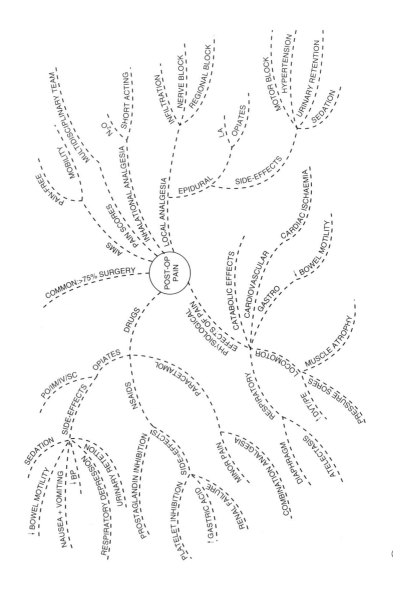

Mind Map®3. Post-operative pain

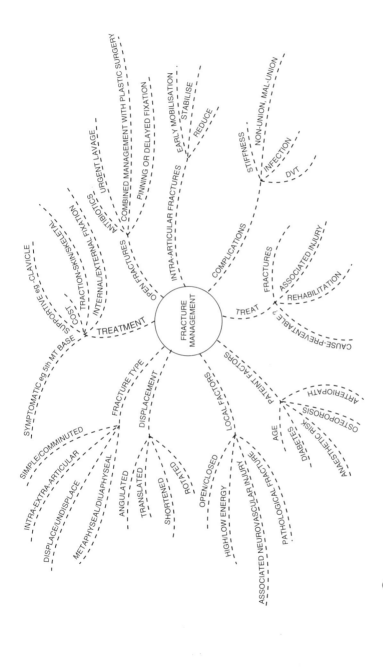

Mind Map®**4.** Fracture Management (reproduced with permission T Branfoot)

Appendix 3:
Useful addresses

The Royal College of Surgeons of England
35–43 Lincoln's Inn Fields
London WC2A 3PN
Tel: 0207 312 6625
Fax: 0207 312 6623
Internet: *www.rcseng.ac.uk*
Application form: *www.rcseng.ac.uk/public/exams/
mrcsremain.htm*

The Royal College of Surgeons of Edinburgh
Nicolson Street
Edinburgh EH8 9DW
Tel: 0131 527 1600
Fax: 0131 557 6406
Internet: *www.rcsed.ac.uk*

The Royal College of Physicians and Surgeons of Glasgow
232–242 St Vincent's Street
Glasgow G2 5RJ
Tel: 0141 221 6072
Fax: 0141 221 1804
Internet: *www.rcpsglasg.ac.uk*

The Royal College of Surgeons in Ireland
123 St Stephen's Green
Dublin 2
Eire
Tel: +353 1 402 2100
Internet: *www.rcsi.ie*

Application form: *www.rcsi.ie/postgrad_education/ examinations/application.html*

The Medicine Publishing Group
The Medicine Publishing Company Ltd
62 Stert Street
Abingdon
Oxon. OX14 3UQ
Tel: 01235 542803
Internet: *www.medicinepublishing.co.uk*

Index

basic science (vivas), 82
enlarged spleen (vivas), 87
gastrointestinal system, 68
neurofibromatosis (vivas), 87
pathology, 24
physiology, 23
rectal bleeding (vivas), 90–1
surgery, 24
multiple choice questions
Crohn's disease, 40
gallstones, 42
ketoacidosis, 45
pancreatitis, 43
phaeochromocytoma, 45
splenectomy, 43
suture materials, 39
thyroid disease, 38

Regulations, exam, 3
Relaxation skills, 14
Resits
number permitted, 5, 7
timing, 104
Results
exams, 101
investigations, 70–1
Revision
breaks from, 12
environment for, 19
last-minute, 14
practice exams, 13
starting, 27
stopping, 32
strategies, 18–24
testing, 12
timetables, 11–12
use of job in, 20, 54
Revision courses (multiple choice questions),
27–8
Role-playing, 23
Royal College of Physicians and Surgeons of
Glasgow, 3
basic training requirements, 8
contact details, 16, 112
exam components, 8–9
marking method, 9
Royal College of Surgeons in Ireland, 3
basic training requirements, 9
contact details, 17, 112
exam components, 10–11
marking method, 10

Royal College of Surgeons of Edinburgh, 3
basic training requirements, 6–7
contact details, 16, 112
distance-learning courses, 28
exam components, 7–8
marking method, 7
Royal College of Surgeons of England, 3
basic training requirements, 4–5
contact details, 16, 112
distance-learning courses, 28
exam components, 5–6
marking method, 5

SELECT courses, 28
Short cases, 5, 8, 9, 11, 60–1; (key points)
61, 75–6
difficulties, 74–5
finishing, importance of, 75
preparation
courses, 66
example questions, 68
mock exams, 64–6
practising cases, 53, 62–3
predicting cases, 64
techniques, 66–9; (summary) 69–70
answering questions, 70, 94–6
diagnoses, 70, 72–3
investigations, 70–2, 73
memory aids, 21–2, 96–9, 105–11
presenting to examiners, 63, 73–4
for general points see also under Clinical
exams
'Sieves'
anatomical, 96
surgical, 97
STEP courses, 28
Stopping revision, 32
Stress, 13
Structure of presentations, 94–6
Study groups, 20, 53
Study leave, 14
Surgical emergencies, 79
'Surgical sieves', 90
Switches in questions, 41–3
Syllabus lists
multiple choice questions, 28
System subjects
multiple choice questions, 29

Techniques
clinical exams, 93–100